Saoussen Chouchene
Rihem Mezrigui
Achraf Amara

Pharmacogenetics of Antiplatelet Agents

Saoussen Chouchene
Rihem Mezrigui
Achraf Amara

Pharmacogenetics of Antiplatelet Agents

Personalized Optimization of Antiplatelet Therapy: Discovering the Power of Pharmacogenetics

ScienciaScripts

Cover image: www.ingimage.com

This book is a translation from the original published under ISBN 978-620-6-72113-0.

Publisher:
Sciencia Scripts
is a trademark of
Dodo Books Indian Ocean Ltd. and OmniScriptum S.R.L publishing group

120 High Road, East Finchley, London, N2 9ED, United Kingdom
Str. Armeneasca 28/1, office 1, Chisinau MD-2012, Republic of Moldova, Europe
Printed at: see last page
ISBN: 978-620-8-13168-5

TABLE OF CONTENTS

INTRODUCTION

Platelets play a key role in primary haemostasis, but they also contribute significantly to pathological clot formation and vessel occlusion. Since myocardial infarction is most often caused by the superimposition of a platelet-rich clot on existing coronary artery disease, antiplatelet agents are essential in the treatment and secondary prevention of acute coronary syndromes (ACS) and during percutaneous coronary intervention (PCI)**[1]**.

The usefulness of antiplatelet agents has been highlighted in several seminal works, which emphasise their importance in preventing cerebral ischaemia due to various pathological processes. Although these drugs are extremely effective from a population point of view in clinical studies, their efficacy in a given patient may vary according to a multitude of factors, mainly linked to genotype**[2]**.

The study of pharmacogenetics makes it possible to optimise drug treatment according to the patient's physiological characteristics. This rapid evolution from "evidence-based medicine" to "precision medicine" is reflected in an increase in the volume of research in this field and in the clinical implementation of its results**[3]**.

The study of genetic variability is difficult because it generally requires the analysis of a large population in order to be sufficiently powerful to find differences in (sometimes) small sub-populations. In the field of cardiovascular medicine in particular, the new antiplatelet drugs have expanded rapidly over the last decade. In this context, our work focuses on the analysis of genetic variants that influence individual responses to antiplatelet drugs.

1. PHARMACOGENETICS

1.1. Definition of pharmacogenetics

Pharmacogenetics has been defined as "... the study of heredity and response to drugs". It is well known that individuals react differently to drug treatment; certain drugs that are effective or well tolerated by some people may be ineffective or toxic for others. By identifying functional polymorphisms in the genome, the aim is to adapt the dosage of certain drugs to each individual and to identify subjects at risk of developing undesirable drug effects **[4]**.

Once a given drug has been administered to the body, it undergoes several stages before being eliminated. It is first absorbed by the body, then distributed to its site of action where it interacts with its target, receptor or enzyme. It is then metabolised and finally excreted. At each of these stages, genetic variations can have a significant influence. Pharmacogenetics is therefore the result of observations indicating clinical variations resulting from variations in drug metabolism due to genetic inheritance **[5]**.

1.2. History and concept

The history of pharmacogenetics began when clinicians observed that the plasma levels of certain molecules administered at standard doses were significantly higher or lower in certain patients, leading to the discovery of the genetic origin of these variations. The term "pharmacogenetics" was coined by Friederich Vogel in 1959 to define a new science applying genetics and pharmacology to study the influence of inheritance on drug response. The first reports of "classic" pharmacogenetic traits were of drug metabolism disorders in which variations in a single drug disposition gene caused a "genetic" response to a drug. abnormal response to medication. These traits behaved like highly penetrant monogenic traits**[6]**.

However, genetic variability in drug response is mainly attributed to complex characteristics involving several genes with compensatory or overlapping roles. As a result, assessing this variability is also more complex. To account for this complexity, pharmacogenetics has evolved into pharmacogenomics, which studies the influence of multiple genes, including relevant pathways and, ultimately, the entire genome (and its products) as they influence drug response. Pharmacogenomics takes into account inherited (germline) and acquired (somatic; in tumours) deoxyribonucleic acid (DNA) variations, in addition to variations in ribonucleic acid (RNA) expression **[7]**.

This new field combines classical pharmacology and genomics, and applies the use of genetic information at both population and patient level to advance drug research and development and to manage drug selection and dosage.

1.3. Principles of genetics and genomics

Genetic polymorphisms can influence the effect of a drug by altering its pharmacokinetics, pharmacodynamics or both (**Figure 1**), which are the two main determinants of inter-individual differences in drug responses. Pharmacokinetics concerns the amount of drug needed to reach its target site in the body, while pharmacodynamics concerns the way in which targets such as receptors, ion channels and enzymes respond to different drugs **[8]**. Genetic polymorphisms in drug transporters and phase 1 drug metabolism enzymes can alter the pharmacokinetic and pharmacodynamic properties of administered drugs, their metabolites, or both at the target site, thereby altering the pharmacokinetics and pharmacodynamics of drugs. which leads to variability in drug responses. In theory, Single Nucleotid Polymorphism(SNP) or sets of closely related SNPs (haplotypes) in genes involved in pharmacokinetic and pharmacodynamic pathways at any stage can affect an individual's overall drug response**[9]**.

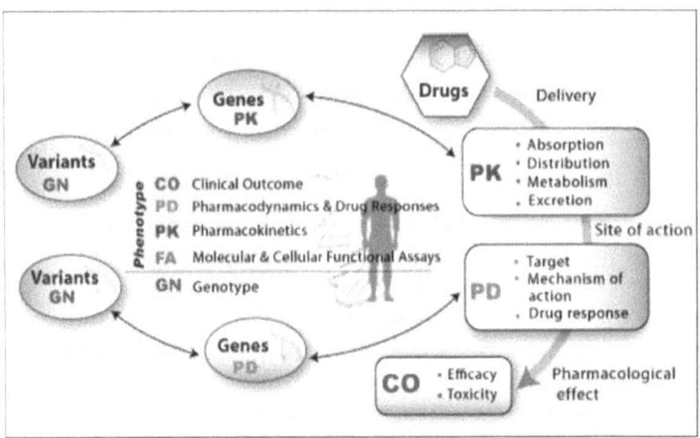

Figure 1: Effect of genetic polymorphisms on the drug response of individuals [10].

CO: Clinical outcome; PD: pharmacodynamic; PK: pharmacokinetics; GN: genotype

1.3.1. Polymorphisms in genes coding for phase I enzymes in drug metabolism

1.3.1.1. Cytochrome P450 2D6

Cytochrome P450 (CYP), a large and diverse group of the heme-containing enzyme superfamily, is involved in the oxidative metabolism of structurally diverse molecules such as drugs, chemicals and fatty acids. Genetic polymorphism in the genes encoding CYP members was first reported for CYP2D6. The highly polymorphic CYP2D6 gene is located on chromosome 22q13.1 and consists of nine exons and eight introns**[11]**.

More than 100 genetic variants of CYP2D6 have been described to date, resulting in point mutations, duplications, insertions or deletions of one or more nucleotides, or even deletions of entire genes. Individuals carrying different CYP2D6 allelic variants have been classified as poor metabolisers (PM), intermediate metabolisers (IM), extensive metabolisers (EM) and ultra-rapid metabolisers (UM) according to the metabolic nature of the drugs and the degree of involvement of these variants in drug metabolism. Although it accounts for only 2 to 4% of the total amount of CYP in the liver, CYP2D6 actively metabolises around 20 to 25% of all drugs administered. Drugs metabolised by CYP2D6 include tricyclic antidepressants, serotonin reuptake inhibitors, antiarrhythmics, neuroleptics and β-blockers**[12]**.

The significant presence of polymorphisms in the CYP2D6 gene significantly affects phenotypic responses to drugs. A difference of up to 10-fold in the dose required to obtain the same plasma concentration has been observed in different individuals. Dextromethorphan, debrisoquine, bufuralol and sparteine are the probe drugs used for in vivo CYP2D6 phenotyping. Depending on the CYP2D6 phenotype, the Caucasian population comprises approximately 5 to 10% of PM, 10 to 17% of IM, 70 to 80% of EM and 3 to 5% of UM**[13]**.

The percentages of PM, IM, EM and UM differ from one ethnic group to another due to the wide variability in the distribution of CYP2D6 alleles.

Individuals with the UM phenotype can metabolise administered CYP2D6 substrates in a much shorter time than individuals with the IM or PM phenotypes. This leads to very low plasma drug concentrations with a potential loss of drug efficacy. Consequently, higher doses of the drug would be required to achieve effective concentrations, which could be fatal in the case of drugs with a narrow therapeutic index. In particular, it has been reported that a large number (around 10 to 30%) of Saudis and Ethiopians have the CYP2D6*2XN allele. On the other hand, individuals carrying the CYP2D6*3, *4, *5 and *6 (PM phenotype) are in the opposite situation. These allelic variants lead to inactive CYP2D6 enzymes, which means that the individuals concerned have high plasma levels of drugs, increasing the risk of side-effects and requiring reduced doses of drugs to be administered**[14]**.

The prodrug tamoxifen is a selective oestrogen receptor (OR) modulator used to treat patients with OR-positive breast cancer. Tamoxifen is actively catalysed to endoxifen and 4- hydroxytamoxifen by various CYPs, with CYP2D6 being the rate-limiting enzyme. Plasma levels of endoxifen in UM patients are generally higher than in PM and IM patients due to the presence of several functional copies of CYP2D6**[15]**.

In patients with RO-positive breast cancer treated with tamoxifen by surgical resection, a significantly lower prevalence of moderate to severe hot flushes, as well as a higher risk of disease relapse, was reported in women with the CYP2D6*4/*4 genotype than in patients with one or no CYP2D6*4 allele (20%). Codeine is a commonly prescribed analgesic which is converted to its active metabolite, morphine, and acts on mu-opioid receptors to induce analgesia. The affinity of morphine for mu-opioid receptors is 200 times greater than that of codeine. Interestingly, the conversion of codeine to morphine is also catalysed by CYP2D6, which has been shown to be the key enzyme responsible for the analgesic effect of codeine. The CYP2D6 phenotype is therefore a determining factor in opioid analgesia. Subjects with the PM phenotype can convert only 10% of a dose of codeine into morphine, whereas this conversion is around 40% and 51% in MEs and UMs, respectively. Therefore, in individuals with CYP2D6 null allelic variants, codeine is not recommended as an analgesic due to minimal enzymatic conversion of codeine to morphine. Conversely, a higher risk of morphine toxicity may occur in patients with the UM phenotype due to the rapid conversion of codeine to morphine. The situation would be even more devastating in UMs who are nursing mothers, as the normal dose of codeine can result in fatal levels of morphine in breast milk. The *10, *17 and *41 allelic variants of CYP2D6 show normal catalytic activity, but are sometimes associated with intermediate or low metabolic activity**[16]**.

1.3.1.2. Cytochrome P450 2C9

According to a number of in vitro studies, carrying one or both of the mutated CYP 2C9 alleles causes a 5-20% reduction in the catalytic activity of these enzymes. Cytochrome P450 2C9 is a hepatic enzyme which metabolises many drugs, including warfarin and other anti-vitamin K drugs (AVKs). Two allelic variants are classically sought, CYP2C9*2 and CYP2C9*3, which show reduced catalytic activity**[17]**.

In the Iranian and Pakistani populations, the prevalence of CYP2C9*2 and CYP2C9*3 is higher than in the other populations. On the other hand, the Chinese, Vietnamese, Korean, Bolivian and Malaysian populations have an allelic frequency of the CYP2C9*1 variant greater than 90%, whereas the CYP2C9*2 allelic variant has not been detected in the Korean, Chinese and Vietnamese populations, but is present at 1% in the Japanese. In addition, no individual from the South African or Zimbabwean populations has been reported to carry the CYP2C9*2 allele**[18]**.

Inter-individual and inter-ethnic variations in CYP2C9 polymorphisms are clinically significant, particularly in patients undergoing anticoagulant treatment with warfarin. Warfarin is one of the most widely prescribed oral anticoagulants. Clinically available warfarin is a racemic mixture of R and S enantiomers, with the S isomer exhibiting approximately 5 times greater anticoagulant potency than the R isomer. Inactivation of active S-warfarin is almost exclusively mediated by CYP2C9. Patients with a high frequency of wild-type CYP2C9 or CYP2C9*1 alleles normally excrete S-warfarin from the body. In contrast, PMs with high allele frequencies of CYP2C9*2, CYP2C9*3, or both, have impaired ability to metabolise S-warfarin and therefore require lower drug doses to achieve therapeutic responses. Thus, PMs have a higher risk of internal bleeding than individuals with a higher CYP2C9*1 allele frequency when treated with warfarin. Although polymorphisms in genes coding for blood coagulation factors also contribute to haemorrhage risk and the need to adjust the initial dose of warfarin, polymorphisms in the CYP2C9 gene still exert a greater influence**[10]**.

1.3.1.3. Cytochrome P450 2C19

Polymorphic CYP2C19, located on chromosome 10q24, codes for another member of the CYP family. CYP2C19 can metabolise many commonly administered drugs, such as anxiolytics (diazepam), proton pump inhibitors (PPIs), anticonvulsants (S-mephenytoin) and antimalarial biguanides. To date, more than 35 CYP2C19 variants and around 2,000 SNPs have been identified, with a steady increase in the number of SNPs reported. Of these, CYP2C19*2 and CYP2C19*3 are the most common variants that have been extensively studied. Both are null variants and patients carrying these variants are therefore classified as PM. CYP2C19*2 is the most common allelic variant, caused by a single nucleotide alteration in exon 5 (G > A), resulting in an abnormal splice site and conferring reduced enzymatic activities to CYP2C19**[19]**.

The CYP2C19*2 variant is present at a high allelic frequency (30%) in South Indians, but at the lowest frequency (2.9%) in the Faroe Islands. In contrast, the CYP2C19*3 variant is present at higher allelic frequencies in Japanese (around

13%) and lower frequencies in Italians, South Africans, Greeks, European-Americans and other populations. Approximately 15-25% of Koreans, Japanese and Chinese have been reported to be PMs of the anticonvulsant S-mephenytoin. The activity of omeprazole, a drug recommended for treating peptic ulcers and gastro-oesophageal reflux disease, has been shown to be highly dependent on patients' CYP2C19 genotypes**[10]**.

1.3.1.4. Cytochrome P450 3A4 and 3A5

More than 2 CYP3A4 SNPs have been described, the most studied of which is the one located in the 5' region of this gene, called CYP3A4*1B. Kidney transplantation studies have shown that people on Tacrolimus (Tac), carriers of the CYP3A4*1B polymorphism, require higher doses and therefore have lower residual tac levels compared with carriers of the wild-type genotype. Another polymorphism, CYP3A4*22, has been shown in studies to be involved in variations in the dose of Tac required. Carriers of this variant show a reduction in hepatic expression of the enzyme in question, leading to a reduction in metabolism in these patients, who run the risk of overdosing and therefore require medium to low doses of Tac**[20]**.
Individuals carrying the CYP3A53 allele have a sequence variation in intron 3 which leads to the creation of a splice site and results in the premature formation of a stop codon, producing a truncated protein. Several studies have demonstrated the association of this CYP3A5 polymorphism with Tac requirements. Patients with a CYP3A51/*1 genotype have high intestinal and hepatic metabolism, requiring a higher daily dose to achieve adequate residual Tac levels. The higher frequency of this allele in the black population could partly explain the less favourable results observed after transplantation. in this population**[21]**.

1.3.2. Polymorphisms in genes coding for transporters of drugs

A drug may have a beneficial or toxic effect on a given patient. The nature and extent of this effect depend largely on the rates of absorption, distribution and excretion of the drug. Drug transporters primarily control the movement of all drugs and their active or inactive metabolites into and out of cells. Consequently, polymorphisms in drug transporter genes can alter the rates of absorption, distribution and excretion and, ultimately, the safety and efficacy of administered drugs. ATP Binding Cassette (ABC) and Solute Carrier (SLC) transporters are two superfamilies of transport proteins that are ubiquitous membrane transport proteins involved in the absorption, distribution and elimination of drugs**[10]**.

ABC transporters often transport drugs and other substances against the concentration gradient using adenosine triphosphate (ATP) as an energy source **[22]**. In the ABC drug transporter superfamily, 49 genes have been identified, which are divided into seven subfamilies, from ABCA to ABCG. The impact of some important polymorphisms on the drug transport activities of various ABC transporters is summarised in **Figure 2**.

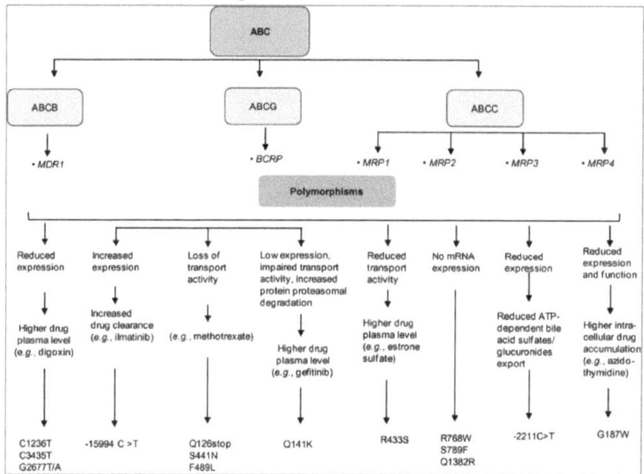

Figure 2: Influence of genetic polymorphisms of adenosine triphosphate Binding Cassette transporters on drug transport activities [10].

ABC: ATP-binding cassette transporter; MDR1: multidrug resistance protein 1; BCRP:breast cancer resistance protein; MRP:multidrug resistance-associated protein.

In addition, around 360 genes have been identified in the SLC superfamily and are classified into 46 subfamilies, among which members of the organic anion transporter, organic anion transporter polypeptide and organic cation transporter subfamilies play a particularly important role in drug elimination. In addition, polymorphisms in the genes encoding members of the SLCO, SLC22 and SLC47 families within the SLC superfamily play a key role in modulating the drug transport activities of the corresponding transporters (**Figure 3**).

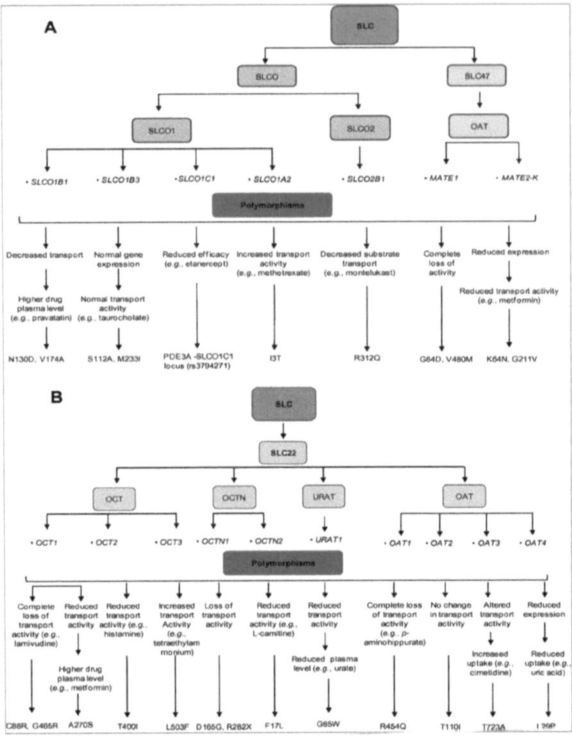

Figure 3: Changes in carriers' drug transport activities solute carrier by genetic polymorphisms [10].

SLC: solute carrier; SLCO: solute carrier organic anion; OCT: organic cation transporter; OCTN: organic cation transporter novel; OAT: organic anion transporter; MATE1: multidrug and toxin extrusion protein 1; URAT: urate transporter.

1.3.3. Polymorphisms in genes involved in variationpharmacodynamics

Pharmacodynamics reflects the ability of a drug to influence its targets, normally a receptor or an enzyme, and can involve both intended and unintended effects. Pharmacodynamic variations include genetic variation in expression levels in the target, as in the case of the human molecular target of warfarin, VKORC1**[23]**.

The VKORC1 gene codes for the VKORC enzyme, a key enzyme in the vitamin K regeneration cycle. It is the pharmacological target of VKAs. This gene contains several genetic polymorphisms, the most extensively studied of which are located in the 1639g>A promoter region, in the 5' non-coding region (VKORC1*2, rs9934438). The latter is in linkage disequilibrium with the VKORC1*intron polymorphism. According to data reported in the literature, carriage of the VKORC1*2 polymorphism causes a reduction in transcriptional activity of around 45%, with subjects carrying this allele requiring lower doses of VKAs than subjects carrying the wild-type allele. The VKORC1 genotype therefore predicts response to VKAs (and therefore the risk of haemorrhage) by explaining 30 to 40% of the variability in acenocoumarol dosage. In Caucasians, the frequency of the mutated A allele is around 43%, and various studies have shown the benefit of genotyping in determining the necessary dosage of VKA before initiating treatment**[24]**.

1.4. The benefits of pharmacogenetics

The main objectives of pharmacogenetic biomarkers are to select the appropriate treatment and dosage for each patient; drugs that are mainly metabolised by a single enzyme should be avoided in poor metabolisers (null alleles), while dosage adjustments can be made in the case of partially reduced or increased activity.However, the predictions of biomarkers of enzyme activity often show considerable variability, even when genomic knowledge is taken into account, which limits their clinical usefulness, as is the case with CYP2D6 variants. Therapeutic decisions must therefore take into account multiple personal factors, including compliance with treatment, which can play an important role, particularly with antipsychotics**[25]**.

The inclusion of pharmacogenetic biomarkers has the potential to reduce adverse events and improve therapeutic outcomes. However, variants present in transporters and receptors, as well as gene networks that affect disease state, introduce confounding factors that are difficult to resolve, limiting clinical utility to specific conditions. The crucial question to be answered is whether the benefits of introducing a biomarker outweigh the additional effort and costs associated with its use. The integration of pharmacogenomic data into electronic medical records, combined with clinical decision support, will be essential for the development of personalised therapy. Access to genetic information is most effective when it is available at the time of drug prescription. Consequently, prospective genotyping of most pharmacogenetic variants or eventually whole genome sequencing are being implemented, but they face logistical problems such as reimbursement, communication of preventive results throughout an individual's life, data portability and privacy protection**[26]**. It is estimated that clinically actionable genotypes for at least one 'pharmacogene' are present in 90-

95% of individuals, yet implementation remains relatively low.A survey in Florida found that only 27% of physicians surveyed used pharmacogenomic information, mainly due to the lack of guidelines or protocols. However, guidelines for the implementation of PGx have been made widely available through national and international consortia**[27]**.

Preventive pharmacogenetic tests with point-of-care decision support are still largely unavailable. A study using a genotyping panel for all "actionable" pharmacogenes, "Implementation of Point-of-Care Pharmacogenomic Decision Support Accounting for Minority Disparities" provides indications for implementation in general practice, particularly for African-American populations, and guidelines for hospital workflows.Pharmacogenetics helps to select the most appropriate drug and dosage to obtain the best therapeutic response. Several clinical guidelines are available for anticoagulants, antiplatelets, transplant drugs and other therapies. Clinical decision-making depends on many factors, such as the patient's genetic variants, the population and quality of the evidence, the availability of tests and pharmacogenetic data, the pharmacokinetics and pharmacodynamics of the drug, the history of the drug and drug interactions. Service providers must also have a good knowledge of pharmacogenetic resources in order to make accurate clinical decisions. Pharmacogenetics contributes primarily to the implementation of personalised medicine by identifying patients who should receive a lower or higher dose, or a different drug. The implementation of pharmacogenetics faces challenges such as clinical testing, data analysis, lack of education and ethical, legal and social implications. Despite these obstacles, several academic, medical and community centres have launched programmes to implement pharmacogenetics. Future advances in precision medicine and data sharing between healthcare providers and patients will help to achieve this goal**[28]**. In addition, genomics has become an integral part of the discovery and development of new drugs for clinical use. The detection of valuable drug targets benefits from the integration of the genomic sequence, transcriptomes of affected tissues, the proteome and the metabolome. For example, genetics has revealed that PCSK9 deficiency protects against cardiovascular disease by reducing cholesterol levels, leading to On the other hand, most common diseases, such as diabetes, cardiovascular disease and psychiatric disorders, have a polygenic origin. In theory, it would be possible to classify these common diseases into subtypes based on their pathophysiology and distinct genetics, but progress in this area has been slow due to the complexity of the network of genes involved. Nevertheless, biomarkers can be used to identify subgroups of patients who would benefit most from specific treatment or who are at increased risk of adverse effects**[25]**.

2. ASPIRIN

2.1. General information on aspirin

2.1.1. History and structure chemical

In the 5ème century BC, Hippocrates made a discovery that extracts from the bark of the white willow tree soothed aches and pains. These extracts were later found to contain salicin, a substance chemically similar to acetylsalicylic acid, better known as aspirin. In 1897, Felix Hoffman succeeded in synthesising aspirin for the first time. Over the course of the 20th century, aspirin became the most widely used medicine in the world. Aspirin is an O-acetyl derivative of salicylic acid (ASA:acetylsalicylic acid) and its main mechanism of action is thought to be the transfer of this acetyl group to salicylic acid**[29]**.
Aspirin is an acronym for acetyl (part of the chemical), spirea (an ornamental plant) and as in salicin (the compound from which aspirin is derived). Aspirin's chemical formula is C H O_{984} **(figure 4)[30]**.

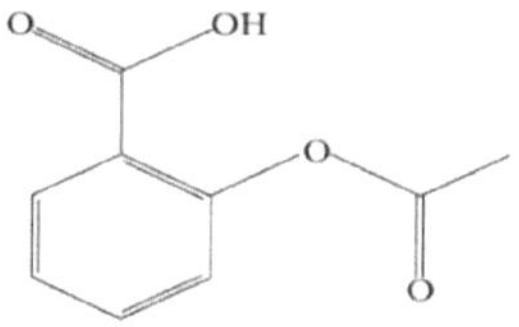

Figure 4: Chemical structure of acetylsalicylic acidC9H8O4[30].

2.1.2. Mechanism of action

In 1971, Vane demonstrated the action of aspirin in inhibiting the synthesis of prostaglandins from arachidonic acid (AA). It acts on a key enzyme: cyclooxygenase (COX), which exists in two isoforms: COX-1 and COX-2. This enzyme, present on the membrane of the reticulum Aspirin is a preferential inhibitor of COX-1, its affinity for COX-1 being 150 to 200 times greater than that for COX-2, which explains the dose-dependent effects of aspirin. When taken in low doses, aspirin acts by irreversibly inhibiting the platelet cyclooxygenase enzyme (COX-1), preventing the conversion of AA to PGH2 and thus inhibiting the production of thromboxane A2 (TXA2) by the thromboxane A2 synthase enzyme (TXA2S) (**Figure 5)[31]**.

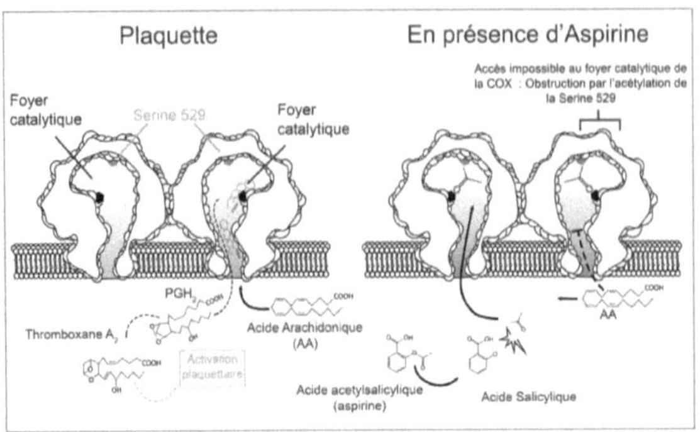

Figure 5: Mechanism of action of aspirin [32].
AA: Arachidonic acid; PGH2: Prostaglandin H2; COX: Cyclo-oxygenase

Pharmacological inhibition of COX-1 begins within a few minutes and maintains the inhibited platelets for their entire lifespan of 7 to 10 days**[32]**.

2.1.3. Pharmacokinetics of aspirin

2.1.3.1. Absorption and bioavailability

Aspirin is absorbed rapidly when taken as a solution, and more slowly when taken as a gastro-resistant tablet. Absorption is rapid in the stomach and upper intestine by the passive route, and peak plasma concentrations of aspirin are generally reached 30 to 40 minutes after ingestion, with TXA2-dependent inhibition of platelet function becoming apparent approximately one hour later. However, when aspirin is administered as an enteric coating, it may take 3 to 4 hours to reach peak plasma concentrations. The bioavailability of single oral aspirin tablets is approximately 40-50% over a wide range of doses**[33]**.

2.1.3.2. Distribution

Aspirin has a volume of distribution of 0.115 to 0.2 L/kg, allowing it to diffuse into most tissues and body fluids. Unlike salicylic acid, aspirin is poorly bound to plasma proteins (around 33% at serum concentrations of 120µg/ml), but it can acetylate serum albumin, thereby interfering with the binding of other molecules, such as phenylbutazone. It should be noted that acetylation of serum albumin is inhibited by salicylate**[34]**.

2.1.3.3. Metabolism

In addition, the COX-1 activity of peripheral platelets is largely inhibited in portal blood, before the first passage to the liver (**figure 6**)**[35]**.

Aspirin undergoes pre-systemic inactivation by deacetylation to salicylic acid by human carboxylesterases (CEs) in plasma and liver. Deacetylated salicylic acid is practically incapable of inhibiting platelet COX-1, and TXA2 generation, when aspirin is administered in low doses. The hepatic isoform 2 of EC (HCE2) mainly accounts for the first-pass hepatic activation of aspirin. HCE2 is also present in the intestine, where it may contribute to the pre-systemic deacetylation of aspirin, before the liver. In addition to HCE2, other ECs are present in the blood, such as cholinesterases, intra-erythrocyte hydrolases and other plasma esterases known as "aspirin esterases" **[35]**.

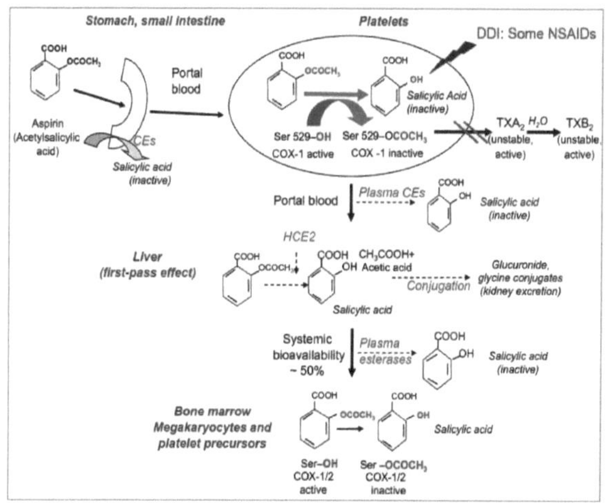

Figure 6: Metabolism of aspirin [35].

CE: carboxylesterases; COX: cyclooxygenase; DDI: drug-drug interaction; HCE2: hepatic isoform 2 of CE;NSAID: non-steroidal antiplatelet drugs;TX: thromboxane.

After hydrolysis, the pharmacokinetics of salicylic acid are characterised by the following:

- A low volume of distribution (0.12 to 0.14 litres/kg) at concentrations therapeutics.
- Strong binding to plasma proteins, particularly albumin.
- Dose-dependent hepatic metabolism for doses below 300 mg. However, at higher doses, the liver's capacity to eliminate salicylic acid is limited, leading to an accumulation of the substance in the body **[34]**.

2.1.3.4. Elimination

Only 1% of an aspirin dose is excreted unchanged in the urine. A small proportion of unmetabolised salicylic acid is eliminated by the kidney, the remainder in the form of inactive metabolites. The plasma half-life of aspirin is 13 to 31 minutes[34].

2.1.4. Indications

2.1.4.1. Primary cardiovascular prevention

The role of aspirin in primary prevention remains uncertain and the subject of debate. In 2018, major studies concluded that there was no benefit from aspirin in terms of the primary prevention of cardiovascular disease. These studies showed an unfavourable benefit/risk ratio, which calls into question the indication of aspirin as a primary prevention measure in individuals with no history of cardiovascular disease or risk factors. In these cases, the risk of bleeding is potentially increased, which limits the use of aspirin for preventive purposes[36].

2.1.4.2. Secondary cardiovascular prevention

❖Acute coronary syndrome

For the treatment of ACS, it is recommended to administer an oral loading dose of aspirin of between 150 and 325 mg, or an intravenous dose of 80 to
The ISIS-2 (International Study of Infarct Survival-2) study formally established the major benefit associated with the use of aspirin within 24 hours of the onset of symptoms of a suspected myocardial infarction (MI) and continued for 5 weeks, with a 23% reduction in mortality and a reduced risk of re-infarction during the period of hospitalisation[37].

❖Ischaemic stroke and transient ischaemic attack

In the United States, guidelines for the secondary prevention of stroke recommend the daily use of aspirin in doses ranging from 75 to 325 mg. However, a Dutch study showed that the secondary prevention of transient ischaemic attacks with a daily dose of 30 mg aspirin produced similar results in terms of efficacy, while causing fewer haemorrhages and adverse effects compared with a dose of 283 mg. In addition, the efficacy of doses lower than 75 mg was confirmed in The European Stroke Prevention Study. This study demonstrated that a daily dose of 50 mg aspirin for 2 years reduced strokes by 18% compared with the group receiving a placebo[37].

2.2. Variability in response to aspirin

Great variability in the pharmacodynamic response to aspirin has been reported. Multiple signalling pathways are involved in platelet activation, and a treatment strategy that inhibits a single pathway may not prevent all thrombotic events. The occurrence of ischaemic events in patients treated with aspirin cannot be attributed to failure of aspirin treatment alone, and failure of treatment alone is therefore not sufficient evidence of resistance to antiplatelet agents**[38]**.

2.2.1. Definition of resistance to aspirin

Inter-individual variability in response to aspirin has been popularised under the term 'aspirin resistance' (AR). However, this term has been inappropriately used to describe a number of heterogeneous phenomena, including aspirin resistance, including the inability of aspirin to :

- Protect individuals from thrombotic complications;
- Prolong bleeding time;
- Reduce production of TXA2;
- Ouproduce a typical effect on in vitro tests of platelet function**[33]**.

This classification, based on new methods, has made it possible to distinguish between different types:

- Type 1 or 'pharmacokinetic', aspirin is ineffective but the addition of aspirin in vitro produces an antiplatelet effect with inhibition of TXA2 formation;
- Type 2 or "pharmacodynamic", neither oral aspirin nor in vitro addition provides an antiaggregant effect;
- Type 3 or "pseudoresistance", platelet aggregation is induced by low concentrations of collagen despite complete inhibition of TXA2 by aspirin**[39]**.

Aspirin resistance can also be classified into biological resistance and clinical resistance:

- Biological resistance' to aspirin is present when the reactivity in vitro is not adequately blocked despite the use of aspirin
- Clinical resistance' to aspirin is defined as the inability to aspirin to prevent clinical atherothrombotic events in patients taking aspirin**[39]**.

2.2.2. Methods for detecting resistance to aspirin

There are currently several methods for testing platelet function, some of which are used in the laboratory (e.g. optical aggregometry, flow cytometry), while others can be used as bedside tests (Innovance PFA-200, VerifyNow Test). The most commonly used platelet function tests are summarised in **Table I**.

Table I: Main common platelet function tests for the detection of aspirin resistance [40].

Platelet test	Test principle	Benefits	Disadvantages
Optical aggregometry(LTA)	Photometry: Evaluation of the variation in light transmission through a platelet suspension (platelet-rich plasma). This transmission increases when platelets are aggregated by an agonist (AA in particular).	-Different platelet pathways analysed using a large number of agonists "gold standard Large number of results from studies on antiplatelet resistance Flexible -Clinical correlation	-Qualified technician required -Large sample volume -Poor reproducibility -Important time
Platelet Function Analyser (PFA)	-Assesses primary haemostasis in whole blood under high shear forces. It records the occlusion time of an orifice in a collagen-coated membrane. Collagen-epinephrine cartridges are highly sensitive to aspirin treatment with lengthening in 88% of cases.	-Easy to use, quick test -Uses whole blood -Reproducible -Highly sensitive in detecting aspirin resistance	-Poor specificity -Sensitive to haematocrit and plasma Von Willebrand factor concentration -Threshold value not defined
VerifyNow	-Fully automated form of optical aggregometry. It measures platelet aggregation using ADP as an agonist and fibrinogen-coated beads. This platelet aggregation is quantified in aspirin reaction unit (ARU).	-Quick and easy test -Uses whole blood -High specificity (0.95) -Reproducible -Sensitivity in aspirin resistance studies with clinical correlation.	- Costly

Table I (continued): Main common platelet function tests for the detection of aspirin resistance [40].

Platelet test	Test principle	Benefits	Disadvantages
Impedance aggregometry	-Impedance: Platelet activation will induce platelet aggregation and adhesion to the electrodes, resulting in an increase in impedance. Platelet aggregation will be quantified by the air under the electrode. aggregation curve [AUC].	- Performed on whole blood -High sensitivity in the detection of aspirin resistance -Simultaneous platelet aggregation test in duplicate for better quality control of each sample	Non-reproducible -High cost
Impact-R	-A whole blood analysis system that applies high shear stress across an acrylonitrile-butadiene-styrene cone to initiate platelet activation and adhesion to a polystyrene well. The well was then washed and stained with May-Grundwald solution. The samples were then analysed using an inverted light microscope connected to an image analyser, and platelet adhesion was determined by examining the percentage of the total surface area covered by platelets (% of surface coverage)	- Quick and easy -Uses whole blood -Reduced sample volume -No sample preparation required	-Expensive

2.2.3. Non-genetic mechanisms involved in aspirin resistance The various mechanisms involved in aspirin resistance are incompletely elucidated. elucidated. Several mechanisms could explain the occurrence of this resistance (**tableII**).

Table II: Main non-genetic mechanisms responsible for aspirin resistance [41].

Intrinsic mechanisms	-Metabolism accelerated by esterases -Alternative pathways of platelet activation : Failure to inhibit platelet activation mediated by catecholamines (epinephrine) Increased regulation of COX-independent pathways (thrombin, TXA2, collagen) -High platelet turnover: surgery, trauma, syndrome myeloproliferative
Extrinsic mechanisms	-Non-compliance with treatment -Inadequate/inappropriate dosage of aspirin -Drug interactions: NSAIDs (ibuprofen); PPIs...

NSAID: non-steroidal anti-inflammatory drug; COX: Cyclooxygenase;PPI: Proton Pump Inhibitor; TXA2: Thromboxane A2

2.2.4. Genetic mechanisms involved in resistance to aspirin

AR has been shown to be largely dependent on polymorphisms in a number of genes (**figure 7**), the main one being the COX-1 gene. SNPs in these genes (C50T, A842G and A1676G) affect the expression of the COX-1 gene and its biological activity**[42]**.

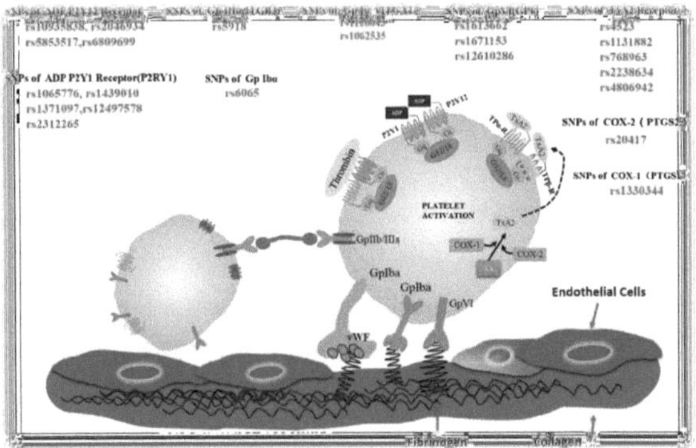

Figure 7: Overview of mediators and genes reported in the literature to influence the antiplatelet effect of aspirin[42].

COX: Cyclooxygenase; TXA2: Thromboxane A2; ADP: Adenosine Di-Phosphate; SNP: Single Nucleotid Polymorphism.

2.2.4.1. Cyclo-oxygenase 1 polymorphism

COX-1 is encoded by the PTGS1 gene, and several polymorphisms of this gene have been studied. Of these, binding imbalance in the C50T polymorphism (rs3842787) has been the most commonly studied as a predictor of reduced aspirin efficacy**[43]**.

Specific variations in PTGS1 appear to regulate AA-induced thromboxane production and platelet aggregation, ultimately affecting the efficacy of this anti-platelet drug, so if they confer increased COX-1 activity, these alterations may contribute to a poor or lack of response to aspirin, ultimately leading to AR.

More specifically, Halushka et al**[44]** reported two SNPs of PTGS1, rs10306114 (A-842G) and rs3842787 (C50T), in complete linkage disequilibrium with each other, which have an impact on AA-induced platelet aggregation. They observed that heterozygous carriers of the haplotype for these two markers showed significantly increased inhibition of expression compared with homozygous individuals ($p = 0.01$). This was consistently observed in patients with cardiovascular disease, notably by observing that carriers of the GCGCC haplotype (-842G) and also carriers of the mutated allele in the signal peptide showed significantly reduced sensitivity to aspirin ($p = 0.009$), as determined by AA-induced platelet aggregation. This study was in agreement with the study developed by Lepäntalo et al **[45]**, in which carriers of the rs10306114 mutated allele showed a poorer response to aspirin ($p = 0.017$). Maree et al**[46]** genotyped144 patients with coronary artery disease on aspirin for five polymorphisms (including A842G, C50T and C22T). Using measurements of thromboaxen B2 (TXB2: a stable product of TXA2 metabolism) and AA-induced platelet aggregometry, the COX-1 haplotype significantly modulated the antiplatelet effect of aspirin. In particular, the A-842G haplotype was associated with a reduced response to aspirin. Similar observations concluded that the C50T polymorphism was not associated with thrombotic events in a study of aspirin-treated patients. Similarly, Lordkipanidzé et al. assessed AA-induced platelet aggregation in patients with aspirin-treated coronary artery disease and found no association with the C22T polymorphism (rs1236913)**[47]**. Another study demonstrated that healthy subjects treated with aspirin and carrying the C50T mutant polymorphism of the COX-1 gene showed a twofold increase in thromboxane production in vivo. Conversely, in the same study, these authors did not find any concordant results for the decrease in sensitivity to aspirin assessed by two different means, namely platelet aggregometry and the PFA-100 automaton. Furthermore, Clappers et al. showed that in a cohort of cardiovascular patients using low-dose aspirin, the COX-1 C50T polymorphism was not associated with a higher risk of atherothrombotic events. This may be due to the fact that the C50T polymorphism is not associated with a higher risk of atherothrombotic events. can be explained by the presence of numerous factors modulating the response to aspirin, it is indeed a multifactorial phenomenon which involves various quite complex genetic, pharmacological, pharmacokinetic and functional mechanisms. Consequently, a single polymorphism is not sufficient on its own to induce such a non-response to aspirin**[48]**. The study by Chakroun et al**[49]** showed no statistically significant association between the C50T polymorphism of the COX-1 gene and non-response to aspirin in patients with stable coronary heart disease. Thus, screening for the C50T polymorphism alone may not be useful for clinical prediction of AR. Overall, despite several studies supporting the association between rs10306114/rs3842787 and a poor response to aspirin, other studies have not confirmed their role in resistance. It is also important to stress that the study of other genes is necessary to trace the relationship between resistance and genetics**[42]**.

2.2.4.2. Cyclo-oxygenase 2 enzyme polymorphism

COX-2, encoded by the PTSG2 gene, has been investigated as a genetic cause of aspirin variability, as it has been found to be expressed in 8-10% of circulating platelets. The C765G polymorphism (rs20417) has been shown to confer reduced COX-2 activity and, interestingly, lower cardiovascular risk; in contrast to studies that have observed an increase in cardiovascular risk with COX-2 inhibition. In an analysis of 49,232 patients, possession of the mutated rs20417 allele reduced the risk of major cardiovascular events (OR: 0.78, 95% CI: [0.70-0.87]). This effect was particularly significant in aspirin users (OR: 0.74, 95% CI: [0.64-0.84]) compared with non-users (OR: 0.87, 95% CI: [0.72-1.06]), indicating that aspirin treatment in this population confers a greater benefit in patients with this polymorphism**[43]**.

Studies have shown that the C765G (rs20417) genetic polymorphism affecting the promoter region of the COX-2 gene is associated with the development of AR, and the mutant allele can upregulate COX-2 expression by altering the promoter**[50]**. The relationship between the COX- 2-(765G> C) gene polymorphism and resistance is controversial in the study by Sharma et al **[51]**, which included 450 patients with ischaemic stroke treated with aspirin, the patients were followed and then divided into two groups, one with a good prognosis and the other with a poor prognosis, and the distribution of the two genotypes was compared. They found that the CC and GC genotypes were associated with adverse vascular events and that patients carrying the C allele were more likely to develop AR than non-carriers. However, Cipollone et al **[52]** have shown that the incidence of cerebral infarction and MI in patients with the CC and GC genotypes is relatively low, which may be associated with the reduced risk of cardiovascular and cerebrovascular disease. In the study by WANG et al, no single nucleotide polymorphism at -C765G has not been associated with AR**[50]**.

2.2.4.3. Glycoprotein IIb/IIIa polymorphism

Glycoprotein IIb/IIIa (GP IIb/IIIa), also known as integrin αIIbβ3, is a complex of integrins present on the surface of platelets. Platelet GP IIb/IIIa receptors bind fibrinogen, a compound involved in platelet aggregation**[42]**.

Genetic polymorphisms in ITGB3, the gene which codes for GP IIIa, have been associated with differential responses to aspirin treatment, probably leading to an increased incidence of thrombotic events. SNP rs5918 leads to the modification of thymidine by cytosine in exon 2, resulting in the substitution of leucine (PlA1) by proline (PlA2) at amino acid 33 of the protein. Studies suggest that the presence of SNP rs5918 may be closely linked to the AR process by reducing the antiplatelet effects of aspirin and, consequently, increasing the risk of recurrent cardiovascular events. In fact, Szczeklik et al **[53]** noted that carriers of the PlA2 allele appear to be more resistant to the action of aspirin than non-carriers ($p = 0.001$).In addition, the results of a large systematic review (including ten studies evaluating rs5918, four in healthy individuals and six in patients with cardiovascular disease) showed that the PlA2 allele was significantly associated with AR in healthy individuals ($P = 0.009$; OR: 2.36; 95% CI: [1.24-4.48]). Furthermore, with LTA, it was possible to observe a correlation between AR and rs5918. This is consistent with the study by Lim et al on a subset of cardiovascular bypass patients receiving aspirin, which showed that carriers of the PlA2 allele had a systematically more impaired response to ASA after surgery than patients homozygous for the PlA1 allele.On the other hand, some studies claim that the reduced response to aspirin could be due to the PlA1 allele or even fail to confirm the relationship between the rs5918 polymorphism and insensitivity to ASA**[42]**.

Carter et al. found that the presence of the PlA2 allele increased the risk of ischaemic stroke in young women. Although Wagner et al. did not show a similar relationship, in a subgroup analysis they showed that the PlA2 allele is associated with a risk of stroke in young women. A study of stroke subtypes showed that the frequency of the PlA2 allele was twice as high in patients with stroke related to large vessel disease compared with the control group.The mechanism leading to an increased risk of thrombosis is not well understood. Thrombin generation is increased by the presence of PlA2, which may trigger the prothrombotic process. Low-dose aspirin does not reduce thrombin production at the site of injury in the presence of the PlA2 allele in healthy individuals; the presence of the PlA2 allele increases epinephrine levels and ADP-stimulated platelet aggregation. Macchi et al. have shown that Some studies have found no significant relationship between the GP IIIa PlA1/A2 genotype and an effect of aspirin in healthy individuals. A meta-analysis showed that carrying the PlA2 gene was not linked to RA. In the study by Derle et al, the entire study group was examined and found a significant association between being a PlA2 carrier and RA. The rate of the PlA2 allele was 14.9% in the aspirin-resistant group and 21.3% in the aspirin-sensitive group. The association between the PlA2 allele and the rate of AR for different doses was examined. When patients using 100 mg and 300 mg aspirin were compared, a significant association was not found between the rate of AR and being a carrier of the PlA2 allele**[54]**.

A meta-analysis found that the PlA1/A2 polymorphism does not predict AR in the laboratory, suggesting that this polymorphism does not affect the antiplatelet effect of aspirin because aspirin has an upstream inhibitory effect on platelets, which may also explain its inability to predict clinical outcomes**[54]**.

2.2.4.4. Von Willebrand factor polymorphism

Von Willebrand factor (vWF) is a multimeric glycoprotein.The prothrombotic effects of vWF are expressed by a receptor formed by GP Ib, IX and V.GP1BA encodes the α subunit of GP Ib, which holds the vWF binding site and appears to be highly polymorphic. In particular, the GP1BA SNP rs6065 (C1018T) has been associated with ischaemic stroke and response to aspirin.Fujiwara et al. reported a negative role for the C allele of rs6065 in aspirin efficacy, due to high platelet aggregation ($p = 0.004$)**[42]**.

The dehuman platelet antigen-2 (HPA-2) polymorphism results in a substitution of threonine for methionine at codon 161 (rs6065; often referred to as Thr145Met). HPA-2 is in a state of binding disequilibrium almost with another polymorphism in the same gene. This latter polymorphism results from a variable number of tandem repeats producing four different GPIbd isoforms in order of decreasing molecular weight (size polymorphism). This size polymorphism is strongly associated with the HPA-2 polymorphism, meaning that alleles with one or two repeats are closely linked to the 161C allele, while three or four repeats are linked to the 161T allele[55].Another polymorphism, the C-5T polymorphism (rs2243093), located in the Kozak sequence five base pairs upstream of the GPIb gene, has been suggested to correlate with susceptibility to stable or acute coronary heart disease in some studies.The C-5T polymorphism has also been associated with increased platelet reactivity by the PFA-100 test in response to collagen and epinephrine in patients on aspirin monotherapy[47].

2.2.4.5. Collagen receptor polymorphism

GP Ia/IIa and GP VI are the main collagen receptors. Polymorphisms related to GP Ia/IIa and GP VI have been suggested to contribute to the attenuation of the antiplatelet effect of aspirin, and in particular rs1126643 (C807T) of the GPIa subunit has been suggested to have a prothrombotic effect and to be related to AR in some studies[56]. However, one meta-analysis did not support a direct association between rs1126643 and coronary heart disease (CHD) or MI; similarly, other analyses found no clinical association between GP VI SNPs and thrombotic events in patients with CHD. Studies have reported an association between rs1671153 and platelet aggregation in patients with foetal loss.but other GP VI SNPs, such as rs1654410, rs1671153, rs1654419, rs11669150, rs1613662 and rs1654431, have not been associated with thrombotic events. were not identified as frequently as rs12610286in the same experimental group[57].

2.2.4.6. Adenosine diphosphate receptor polymorphism Platelet activation by ADP relies on the stimulation of two purinergic G protein-coupled receptors present on the platelet surface: P2Y1 and P2Y12.The genes encoding P2Y1 and P2Y12 are located on chromosome 3. Polymorphisms in the P2Y1 and P2Y12 loci have been suggested to contribute to a reduction in the antiplatelet effect of aspirin[47].

❖ P2Y1 receptor polymorphism

ADP is an important mediator of platelet function. Fontana et al. propose that genetic polymorphism of the P2Y1 receptor may also contribute to AR.Jefferson et al, examined four genes encoding GPIIIa, COX-1, COX-2 and P2Y1 in 332 patients with a history of MI. They found that AR was significantly associated with the P2Y1 gene C893T. Heterozygous patients were almost three times more resistant to aspirin compared with homozygous patients[58].Jefferson et al [59] studied 469 patients with a history of MI and used aggregometry with AA as an agonist to assess the antiplatelet effect of aspirin.They reported that the T allele of the C893T P2Y1 polymorphism (rs1065776) was significantly associated with a reduced antiplatelet effect of aspirin. In contrast, several studies reported that the T allele conferred an increased platelet response to aspirin and that CC homozygosity was associated with a reduced antiplatelet effect in a Chinese population. This discrepancy highlights the importance of pharmacogenetic variability from one population to another. Others have found that the A1622G polymorphism (rs701265) in the same gene affected platelet response to ADP, but no association of this polymorphism with response to aspirin has been reported in other studies using platelet aggregometry**[47]**.

❖**P2Y12 receptor polymorphism**

Some authors have reported that AR is associated with P2Y12 polymorphisms: Timur et al**[60]** reported the association of P2Y12 polymorphisms with platelet reactivity to aspirin as assessed by LTA and TXB2 in 423 patients with CAD, showing that P2Y12 SNP rs7634096 was associated with low residual platelet reactivity.

2.2.4.7. PEAR1 receptor polymorphism

Platelet endothelial aggregation receptor-1 (PEAR1) is a platelet transmembrane protein that plays an important role in platelet reactivity and endothelial function. The PEAR1 gene comprises 23 exons and 22 introns. The role of PEAR1 polymorphisms in platelet aggregation has been demonstrated in a number of studies, some of which have shown that in patients treated with aspirin, carriers of the A allele of rs12041331 in the PEAR1 gene had a significantly increased risk of MI compared with their GG counterparts. Meta-analyses have shown that the A allele of rs12041331 is associated with reduced platelet aggregation and increased platelet activation in coronary artery disease**[61]**.

Genome-wide association studies (GWAS) identified that a variant in intron 1 of the PEAR1 gene (rs12566888) was associated with ADP- and epinephrine-induced aggregation, and that the rs12566888T allele was associated with a decreased aggregation response. Another variant (rs12041331) in intron 1 was in close linkage disequilibrium with rs12566888, and the G allele was reported to be associated with greater platelet reactivity in the presence and absence of aspirin treatment in African Americans.However, in other studies, no association was observed between platelet activity during aspirin treatment and rs12566888 and rs12041331**[62]**.

2.2.4.8. Thromboxane A2 receptor polymorphism

The TXA2 receptor is a protein which, in humans, is encoded by the TBXA2R gene, and is widely distributed in different cell types and organ systems. SNPs affecting the TXA2 receptor gene affect the risk of developing cerebral ischaemia and platelet function, in particular platelet aggregation. A significant difference in the distribution of rs768963 between patients suffering from cerebral ischaemia and control groups was reported in a Chinese population.however, no significant association was noted between rs4523 variants and cerebral infarction.A study of 110 healthy Japanese individuals examined the association between genetic polymorphisms and the antiplatelet effect of aspirin. The results revealed that alleles 1018C and 924T (rs4523) are likely to be involved in AR**[63]**.The results of various studies on the impact of genetic polymorphisms on response to aspirin are summarised in **Table III**.

Table III: Impact of genetic polymorphisms on the clinicobiological response to aspirin

Study	Method	Sick	Number of patients	Polymorphism/gene studied	Results
Xu et al.2019 [64]	LTA	SCA	2439	PEAR1	The 30-day incidence of major cardiovascular events was significantly higher in AA homozygotes than in non-AA homozygotes (p=0.026), platelet aggregation induced by ADP was significantly lower in AA homozygotes than in non-AA homozygotes (p=0.026), and platelet aggregation induced by ADP was significantly lower in AA homozygotes than in non-AA homozygotes (p=0.026). in GG homozygotes.
Wang et al.2018[50]	PFA	Ischemic stroke	97	COX-2 -765G>C GPIa 807C>T	The analysis showed that the CT+TT genotype at the 807C>T locus was significantly correlated with resistance after adjustment for confounding factors (p=0.047). There were no significant differences in genotype distribution and allele frequency at the COX-2 gene site -765G>C between the two groups (p> 0.05).
Xue et al.2017[65]	LTA	Unstable angina	207	COX-1rs5911rs3842788	There is evidence for the first time that rs5911 and rs3842788 are independently associated with RA in Chinese patients, with a 4.5-fold and 8.3-fold increased risk. respectively.

Table III (continued): Impact of genetic polymorphisms on the clinicobiological response to aspirin

Study	Method	Sick	Number of patients	Polymorphism/gene studied	Results
Yi et al.2016 [66]	LTA	AVC ischemic	850	COX-1COX-2	Individual patients with the combination of rs3842787(CT) and rs20417(CC) or rs3842787(CT) and rs20417(GC) had a significantly higher risk of AR+ AR than those with rs3842787CC and rs20417(GG). High-risk interactions between rs3842787 and rs20417 were independent predictors of AR+ AR, and were associated with a smaller reduction in the risk of AR+ AR. platelet aggregation activity.
Abderrazek et al.2010 [67]	PFA-100	SCA	188	GPIIIa PlA	High platelet reactivity (HPR) patients with inadequate aspirin inhibition were significantly more likely to be PlA1/A1 homozygous (65.4% versus 47.7%, p=0.015). After multivariate analysis, the PlA1/A1 genotype was the only independent risk factor for RPH. persistent (p=0.016).

LTA: Light Transmission Aggregometry;PFA: Platelet Function Analyzer;ACS: acute coronary syndrome;CVA: stroke; AR: aspirin resistance;ARS: aspirin semiresistance;HPR: high platelet reactivity

2.2.4.9. MicroRNAs involved in aspirin resistance

MicroRNAs (miRNAs) are non-coding RNAs that affect post-transcriptional events by inhibiting mRNA translation or inducing mRNA degradation. Platelets have been shown to be involved in specific miRNA patterns. A study using healthy human platelets characterised 532 miRNAs, with the most abundant miRNAs being members of the let-7 family. They are associated with the regulation of P2Y12 and other receptors, affecting the ability of platelets to activate and aggregate. The profile of platelet miRNAs, including miR-223, miR-191, miR-126 and miR-150, has been shown to respond to aspirin treatment. A study from healthy individuals showed that lower expression of miR-19b-1-5p is associated with platelet insensitivity to aspirin, and miR-19b-1-5p expression is a marker for identifying patients at high risk of recurrence **[68]**.

2.3. Aspirin resistance and its consequences

Two case series in stable patients with cardiovascular disease demonstrated an increased risk of major cardiovascular events associated with a poor response to aspirin. Stable patients who had been taking aspirin (325 mg/day) for 7 days were tested for aspirin sensitivity using LTA. A poor response to aspirin was present in 5.2% of patients. After a mean follow-up period of 1.9 years, poor response to aspirin was associated with an increased risk of death, MI or cerebrovascular events compared with aspirin-sensitive patients (24% versus 10%). In a second study, the VerifyNowa aspirin test was used to determine aspirin responsiveness in patients taking aspirin 81-325 mg/day for 4 weeks. A poor response to aspirin was observed in 128 patients (27.4%). After a mean follow-up period of 379 days, patients with a poor response to aspirin had an increased risk of death, MI, stroke, cardiovascular accident and stroke. transient ischaemic attack or unstable angina requiring hospitalisation compared with aspirin-sensitive patients (15.6% versus 5.3%)**[69]**.

In addition, a case-control study measured urinary concentrations of 11-dehydro-thromboxane B2 in patients treated with aspirin as part of the HOPE (Heart Outcome Prevention Evaluation) trial. After five years of follow-up, patients whose levels were in the highest quartile had a mortality rate 1.8 times higher than those in the lowest quartile. Similarly, other studies have reported that incomplete suppression of thromboxane production, as measured by a high concentration of 11-dehydro-thromboxane B2 in urine, is an independent and potentially modifiable determinant of clinical outcomes in patients at risk of aspirin-induced atherothrombotic events. Using PFA-100 to measure aspirin-mediated platelet inhibition, several studies have also reported increased event rates in patients with poor aspirin response profiles. Finally, a meta-analysis involving 15 to 20 studies and nearly 3,000 patients showed that patients identified as having a poor response to aspirin had an almost four-fold increased risk of recurrent cardiovascular events compared with aspirin-sensitive patients. Although the studies included in the meta-analysis were heterogeneous in their methodology, this analysis indicates an association between laboratory-defined poor response to aspirin and adverse clinical events**[70]**.

2.4. Strategy in the event of resistance to aspirin

Some authors suggest trying a higher dosage of aspirin to produce the effect and "break up" RA. Since the degree of inhibition of COX-1 activity depends mainly on the dose of ASA. As part of the long-term prophylaxis of cardiovascular events, lower doses of aspirin are recommended, although this may lead to a more frequent occurrence of AR in the laboratory. Some researchers believe that the administration of of higher doses of aspirin, but only in patients in the acute phase of stroke, may make it possible to "break" the AR detected when lower doses of the drug are used. On the other hand, it should be mentioned that the results of the vast majority of studies do not prove the existence of a relationship between aspirin dose and AR. On the other hand, a higher dose of aspirin is associated with gastrointestinal adverse effects**[71]**. Another proposed solution is the use of dual antiplatelet therapy, i.e. the addition of a second antiplatelet drug to aspirin, generally clopidogrel (at a dose of 75 mg). However, it has been shown that adding clopidogrel to aspirin does not reduce the risk of another cerebrovascular event. The disadvantage of this strategy is also undoubtedly the fact that the use of such therapy, especially for a period of more than 3 months, is associated with a higher risk of haemorrhage, including potentially fatal intracranial haemorrhage. Therefore, it is currently accepted that the best intervention is to replace aspirin with another antiplatelet drug, although the available evidence suggests that this is not an ideal solution**[71]**.

Studies have demonstrated the efficacy of new P2Y12 receptor inhibitors such as ticagrelor, which are already being used successfully in patients suffering from MI. The SOKRATES**[72]** study showed that ticagrelor (at a dose of 2 x 90 mg) was more effective than ASA in inhibiting stroke recurrence, while also reducing the risk of mortality at 3 months post-stroke, particularly in patients with ipsilateral carotid stenosis. The PEGASUS-TIMI**[73]** study showed that the addition of ticagrelor to ASA significantly reduced the risk of another cerebrovascular event without increasing the risk of haemorrhage.

3. ADENOSINE DIPHOSPHATE RECEPTOR INHIBITORS (P2Y12)

3.1. Thienopyridines

3.1.1. Ticlopidine

Ticlopidine, 5-[(2-chlorophenyl)methyl]-4,5,6,7-tetrahydrothieno[3,2-c]pyridine hydrochloride, was approved for use in the United States in 1991**[31]**.
Ticlopidine blocks ADP-mediated platelet aggregation, which decreases the expression of glycoprotein IIb/IIIa via the P2Y12 receptor. When platelets are activated, they secrete ADP, which plays a role in platelet activation and blood clot formation. By preventing the expression of glycoprotein IIb/IIIa and inhibiting fibrinogen binding, Ticlopidine hinders clot formation **[74]**. It is currently rarely used, largely due to the risk of serious side-effects, and consequently no pharmacogenetic studies have been carried out to predict platelet response to this molecule.

3.1.2. Clopidogrel

3.1.2.1. Chemical structure

Clopidogrel or (S)-methyl α-(4,5,6,7-tetrahydrothieno[3,2-c]pyridin-5-yl)- α-(o-chlorophenyl) acetate) is an oral platelet anti-aggregant with a thienopyridine structure(**figure8**).
It has an asymmetric carbon atom in position 7, the configuration of which determines its biological activity. Of the two stereoisomers of clopidogrel available, only the dextrorotatory (S) isomer has antithrombotic and platelet-aggregating effects, while the laevorotatory (R) isomer has no therapeutic effects. Currently, clopidogrel is a racemic mixture made up of two enantiomers in equal quantities. It is marketed in bisulphate form with the following chemical formula: C H CINO$_{16162}$ **S[75]**.

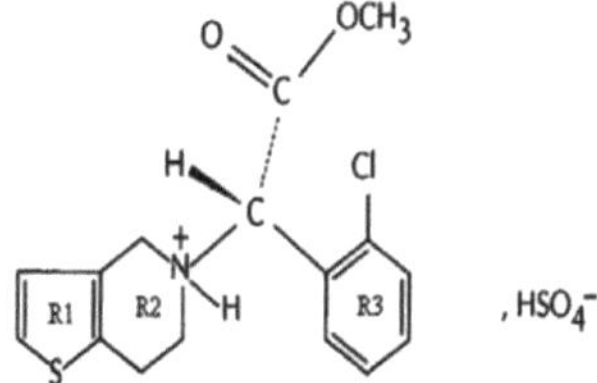

Figure 8: Chemical structure of (S)-clopidogrel bisulphate [75].

3.1.2.2. Mechanism of action

Thienopyridines are structurally related drugs that selectively inhibit ADP-induced platelet aggregation by blocking the P2Y12 receptor. Clopidogrel is a prodrug that must be metabolised by the hepatic CYP P450 enzyme system to acquire activity. Consequently, their onset of action is delayed unless loading doses are administered**[76]**.The active metabolite of clopidogrel exerts inhibition on the platelet P2Y12 receptor activation pathway by ADP, (**figure9**). In the absence of clopidogrel, activation of the P2Y12 receptor leads to the release of Gi protein subunits. This leads to inhibition of adenylate cyclase and a decrease in the concentration of cyclic adenosine monophosphate (cAMP) in platelets. This decrease in cAMP leads to reduced phosphorylation of protein kinase A and dephosphorylation of vasodilator-simulated phosphoprotein (VASP), which promotes activation of the fibrinogen receptor and platelet aggregation.In addition, the B subunit activates phosphoinositol 3-kinase (PI3K) and phosphotyrosine kinase (PI3K), stimulating the secretion of platelet granule contents, including dense granules containing Ca2+, ADP, ATP and serotonin. This activation also promotes activation of the fibrinogen receptor αIIβ3 (GPIIb/IIIa) on platelets**[77]**.

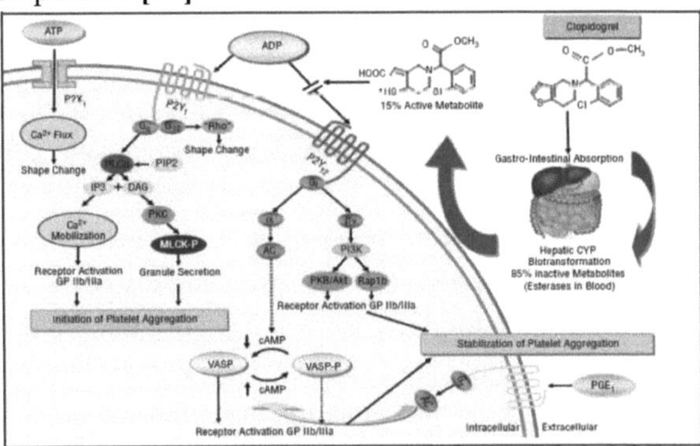

Figure 9: Mechanism of action of clopidogrel [78].

ATP:Adenosine triphosphate; ADP:adenosine diphosphate; PLC:PhospholipaseC; PIP2: Phosphatidylinositoldisphosphate; IP3:Inositol triphosphate; DAG:Diacylglycerol; PK: Protein kinase; MLCK-P:Phosphorylation of myosin light chain kinase; GP:Glycoprotein; AC:Adenylate cyclase; cAMP:Cyclic adenosine monophosphate; VASP: Vasodilator-stimulated phosphoprotein; PI3K: Phosphatidylinositol 3-kinase; PGE1:Prostaglandin E1

3.1.2.3. Pharmacokinetics

❖ **Resorption and distribution**

Clopidogrel is rapidly absorbed and is not strongly affected by food. Clopidogrel is a substrate for P-glycoprotein (P-gp), an ATP-dependent pump responsible for the transmembrane efflux of many drugs. P-gp belongs to the ABC transporter superfamily and is encoded by the MultiDrug Resistance MDR1 (ABCB1) gene. The polymorphism affecting this gene may be responsible for the variability in intestinal absorption of clopidogrel. Clopidogrel and its main circulating metabolite are reversibly bound to plasma proteins (98% and 94% respectively). Distribution is fairly limited. It is restricted to the circulatory system, liver, kidneys, lungs and adipose tissue.were observed approximately 1 hour after administration of a 600 mg loading dose**[79]**.

❖ **Metabolism**

Clopidogrel is a prodrug that requires complex bioactivation via hepatic metabolism involving various drug-metabolising enzymes. Clopidogrel is extensively metabolised, mainly (approximately 85%) by carboxylesterase 1 (CES1) to an inactive carboxylic acid derivative representing the most abundant metabolite in the blood. Approximately 15% of absorbed clopidogrel is biotransformed to its active metabolite by a two-step enzymatic process. In the first stage, clopidogrel is transformed into an inactive intermediate, 2-oxo-clopidogrel, and then in the second stage, transformed into the active thiol metabolite in the presence of reduced glutathione (GSH) (**figure10**)**[79]**.

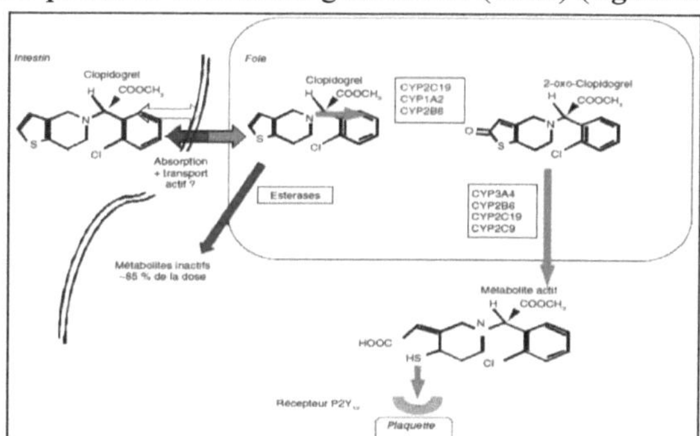

Figure 10:Absorption and metabolism of clopidogrel [77].

Controversial data exist on the enzymes catalysing the formation of the active metabolite. Several in vitro and in vivo studies have indicated CYP2C19 as the main enzyme responsible for clopidogrel bioactivation with CYP1A2, CYP2B6,

CYP2C9, and CYP3A4/5 playing a minor role. However, others suggest that 2-oxo-clopidogrel is mainly formed by intestinal CYP3A4/5 and then metabolised to the active form by paraoxonase 1 (PON 1) **[79]**.

❖ **Elimination**

The active metabolite has a short half-life of about 30 minutes, whereas the half-life of the parent compound is about 6 hours. After a radiolabelled oral dose, approximately 50% of the total radioactivity was found in the urine and faeces respectively**[79]**.

3.1.2.4. Indications

Compared with aspirin in patients with recent ischaemic stroke, MI or peripheral arterial disease, clopidogrel reduced the risk of cardiovascular death, MI and stroke by 8.7%.In some patients, clopidogrel and aspirin are combined to capitalise on their ability to block complementary platelet activation pathways. For example, the combination of aspirin and clopidogrel is recommended for at least 4 weeks after implantation of a bare-metal stent in a coronary artery and for at least 1 year in those with a drug-eluting stent**[76]**.

The combination of aspirin and clopidogrel has also found its place in the prevention of atherothrombotic and thromboembolic events in patients with atrial fibrillation who cannot be treated with anticoagulants, as described by the ACTIVE (Atrial fibrillation Clopidogrel Trial with Irbesanan for prevention of Vascular Events) clinical trial**[80]**.

The combination of clopidogrel and aspirin is also effective in patients suffering from unstable angina. In 12562 such patients, the risk of cardiovascular death, MI or stroke was 9.3% in those randomised to receive the combination of clopidogrel and aspirin and 11.4% in those who received aspirin alone, representing a relative risk reduction of 20%.beneficial in stroke, with a 3.8% reduction in the risk of recurrence without compromising the risk of haemorrhage**[76]**.

3.1.2.5. Variability in response to clopidogrel

The definition of clopidogrel resistance (CR) is inconsistent in the literature for several key reasons. Firstly, there is inconsistency in the terminology attributed to the measurable clinical outcome of undesirably high platelet reactivity despite regular antiplatelet therapy. Terms such as elevated platelet reactivity on treatment, unresponsiveness, and resistance have been used in trials, reviews and meta-analyses to describe an elevated platelet reactivity measurement or an ischaemic clinical outcome despite antiplatelet therapy. These terms are often used interchangeably. The term "antiplatelet resistance" refers to that which results in elevated antiplatelet reactivity or is associated with adverse ischaemic clinical outcomes**[81]**.

Some patients are classified as "poor responders", i.e. they retain little or no change in their platelet aggregation capacity to ADP on clopidogrel compared with baseline, whether by the platelet aggregation test, the VASP test or the VerifyNow P2Y12 test.Despite the heterogeneity of the results, biological resistance to clopidogrel, observed in approximately 20% of patients treated with 75 mg/d of clopidogrel, was associated with an increased risk of cardiovascular events (OR:8; 95% CI:[3.4-19] **[77]**.

3.1.2.6. Non-genetic mechanisms predictive of biological non-response to clopidogrel

Variation in the platelet inhibitory effects of clopidogrel has been shown to be associated with genetic factors, including polymorphisms and epigenetics. However, these data on genetic variation are insufficient to explain variation in response to clopidogrel. There are also other non-genetic factors (**TableIV**), such as demographic characteristics, concomitant diseases and drug interactions influencing the antiplatelet effect of clopidogrel.

Table IV: Non-genetic factors in response variability to clopidogrel [82].

Intrinsic mechanisms	-Inappropriate dose of clopidogrel -Drug interactions between clopidogrel and associated treatment: Clopidogrel and PPIs;Clopidogrel and statins;Clopidogrel and calcium channel blockers -Reduced bioavailability of clopidogrel : Poor compliance; Accelerated metabolism
Extrinsic mechanisms	Age; Sex; Smoking Medical history: Obesity; Diabetes mellitus insulin; Hypertension; Chronic kidney disease... Platelet turnover

PPI: proton pump inhibitors

3.1.2.7. Genetic mechanisms predictive of biological non-response to clopidogrel

There are several identified genetic variabilities that contribute to clopidogrel non-responsiveness. In fact, variable platelet reactivity to clopidogrel is highly heritable. As clopidogrel undergoes intestinal absorption, bioactivation by CYP450 enzymes and deactivation by esterases, this process could be affected by several genetic variants. Genetic variants that could interfere with the variable platelet reactivity of clopidogrel include polymorphisms ofCYP2C19, CYP3A4/5, CYP2C9, BABCB1, PON1, CES1, and the genetic polymorphism of P2Y12 receptors**[83]**.

❖ **Genetic polymorphism affecting intestinal absorption**

The ABCB1 gene codes for the intestinal transporter of multidrug-resistant P-glycoprotein-1, a modulator of clopidogrel absorption. and function, having a direct influence on the systematic availability of its substrates. This variability is partly due to the various genetic polymorphisms affecting the ABCB1 gene. Although it is a silent polymorphism, not leading to changes in the amino acid sequence, C3435T located in exon 26 has been associated with variations in intestinal expression and function of P-gp**[84]**.

In the literature, the involvement of the ABCB1 C3435T polymorphism in CR is controversial.On the one hand, several teams have concluded that there is no significant association between ABCB1 variants and CR, and Su et al**[85]** reported that ABCB1 3435C>T was not associated with CR (p=0.288) in Chinese patients with ischaemic stroke treated with clopidogrel. Also, Li et al**[86]** found that ABCB1 3435C>T SNPs were not associated with CR and recurrent ischaemic events in 268 Chinese patients who had received an extra- or intracranial stent. On the other hand, other studies have demonstrated the involvement of this polymorphism in the reduced responsiveness to clopidogrel and in the occurrence of cardiovascular events.In fact, analysis of the concentration-time curve for clopidogrel and its active metabolite revealed that after a loading dose of 300mg or 600mg of clopidogrel, the Cmax and AUC levels of clopidogrel and its active metabolite were lower in patients carrying the 3435TT genotype compared with patients carrying at least one normal "C" allele. These lower Cmax and AUC values observed in 3435TT carriers suggest increased intestinal efflux, probably as a result of overexpression of P-gp**[87]**.

In addition, Kim et al found that the ABCB1 SNP 3'UTR A>G (rs3842), but not the ABCB1 SNP -154T>C, was associated with the development of ischaemic stroke in a Korean population, in a case-control study,which included 121 participants with ischaemic stroke and 291 control participants**[88]**.

❖ Paraoxonase-1 gene polymorphism

PON1 encodes a protein esterase found mainly in hepatocytes and with a role in regulating high-density lipoprotein homeostasis.PON1 has been described as a key enzyme in the biotransformation of clopidogrel into a more active drug, with two main polymorphisms identified: rs662 (or Q192R) and rs854560 (or L55M)**[43]**.

The data in the literature are convergent. In fact, the study conducted by Bouman et al. revealed a significant association (p=0.001) between the PON1 Q192R genetic polymorphism and the frequency of stent thrombosis at 12 months in patients treated with clopidogrel**[89]**.

In addition, the increased enzymatic activity of PON 1 leads to increased production of the endometabolite from 2-oxo-clopidogrel at the expense of formation of the active metabolite via CYP2C19, which results in a poor response to clopidogrel and therefore a higher risk of thrombosis after PCI.In contrast, Mega et al.reported that the Q192R genetic variant was not associated with pharmacological or clinical response to clopidogrel, and their meta-analysis of 13 studies also showed no statistically significant association between the 192Q variant andMACEs (Major Adverse Cardiovascular Events) during clopidogrel treatment**[90]**.

In addition, the work of Dansette et al. showed that the second stage of enzymatic conversion depends mainly on the cytochrome P450 pathway to convert 2-oxo-clopidogrel to cis 4b, but also depends on PON1 to convert it to the minor "endo" metabolite 4b, whose antiplatelet activity has not yet been determined. These results suggest that the role of PON1 in CR may not be important**[91]**.

❖ Genetic polymorphism affecting clopidogrel metabolism

The cytochromes P450 most involved in the metabolism of clopidogrel to active thiol are CYP3A4 and CYP2C19. Their expression and activity are very The CYP2C19 gene is highly polymorphic, with more than 2000 genetic variants described (**figure 11**), the majority of which are intronic and the minority variants in the coding region**[92]**.

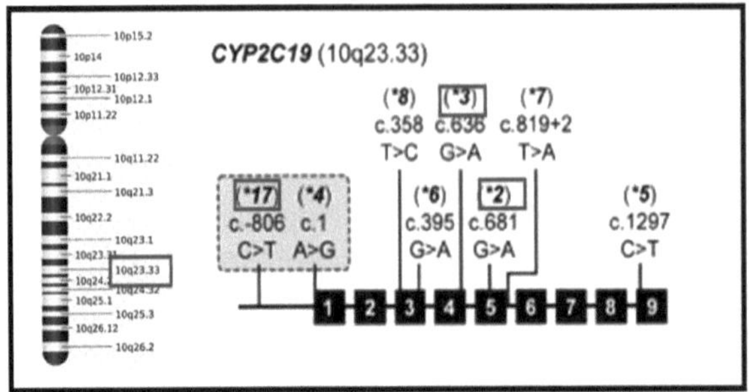

Figure 11: Polymorphisms in the cytochrome P2C19 gene [93].

CYP2C19*2 and CYP2C19*3 are associated with a partial or total reduction in enzymatic activity depending on whether the genotype is homozygous (slow metabolisers) or heterozygous (intermediate metabolisers) and CYP2C19*17 allows ultra-rapid metabolism in the absence of the*2 and *3 alleles. (tableV)[94].

Table V: Metabolic phenotypes according to cytochrome P2C19 genotype [94].

Phenotype	Genotype	Enzymatic activity
Ultra-fast metabolisers (UM)	*1/*17 *17/*17	Normal enzyme activity or enhanced
Extensive metabolisers (EM)	*1/*1	Normal enzyme activity
Intermediate metabolisers (IM)	*1/*2 *1/*3 *2/*17	Intermediate enzyme activity
Slow metabolisers (PM)	*2/*2 *3/*3 *2/*3	Weak or absent enzyme activity

The most commonoss-of-function (LOF) alleles are CYP2C19*2 and *3, which result in degraded or non-functional proteins. The CYP2C19*2 haplotype contains a variant (c.681G>A) which leads to a premature stop codon producing a non-functional protein. The frequency of the minor allele of this single-nucleotide polymorphism varies according to ethnic origin**[92]**.

Carriers of the LOF CYP2C19 allele (PM and IM) have a reduced capacity for clopidogrel bioactivity. A 32% relative reduction in plasma concentrations of the active metabolite has been reported in LOF carriers following exposure to clopidogrel. Consistent with this, the LOF genotype is associated with elevated platelet reactivity during treatment after PCI, which is an independent risk factor for MACEs. Therefore, it follows that LOF carriers treated with clopidogrel may be at greater risk of MACEs after PCI than non-carriers**[95]**.

The presence of LOF CYP2C19 has been associated with high platelet reactivity (HPR) during clopidogrel treatment. In a meta-analysis of 4 studies involving 4341 subjects who received a 600 mg loading dose of clopidogrel, there was a significant residual HPR which appeared to reflect a gene-dose effect in CYP2C19*2 carriers compared with non-carriers (**figure12**).

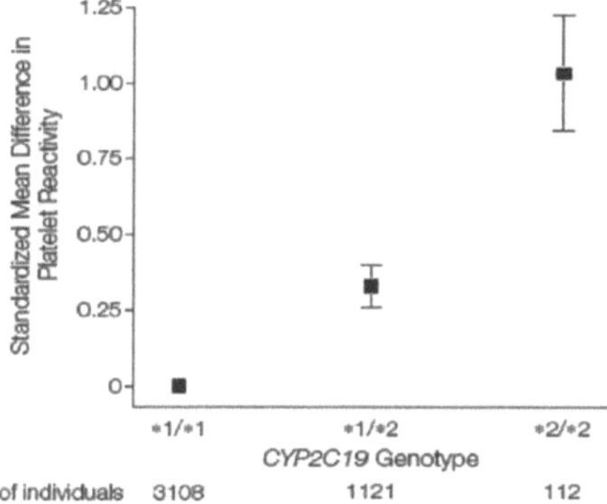

Figure 12: Platelet reactivity according to cytochrome P2C19 genotype after clopidogrel loading [92].

Furthermore, in 2018, an analysis in the haematology department of the Fattouma Bourguiba Hospital in Monastir of 150 coronary patients suggested that carriage of the CYP2C19*2 polymorphism could be a potential predictor of persistent HRP on clopidogrel in diabetics (OR=4.437; p=0.032) whereas this polymorphism had no impact in non-diabetic subjects (p=0.759).This may be explained by several factors. Firstly, diabetes induces an increase in esterase activity, which may lead to a reduction in the generation of the active metabolite of clopidogrel. This decrease is further exacerbated by the presence of the CYP2C19*2 genetic variant, which may lead to an ineffective response to treatment in diabetic patients.In addition to this explanation, other factors may contribute to this poor response, such as increased platelet turnover. This may result in a pool of platelets that have not been exposed to the active metabolite of clopidogrel long enough, particularly during the nocturnal period. It is also important to note that platelets in diabetic patients are often hyperactive, which may require a higher degree of inhibition to achieve an optimal treatment effect**[96]**.

The study by Song et al**[97]** is particularly interesting: it was carried out on 20 healthy volunteers who received 300 mg of clopidogrel and were classified into

3 groups according to genotype: CYP2C19*1/*1 (NM or EM; n=8), CYP2C19*1/*2 or *1/*3 (IM; n=10) and CYP2C19 *2/*2, *3/*3 or *2/*3 (PM; n=2). The study showed a significant impact of CYP2C19*2 and CYP2C19*3 polymorphisms on the pharmacokinetic parameters of clopidogrel (C_{max} and AUC0-t of the active metabolite of clopidogrel) and on platelet reactivity (**figure13**), as well as a significant association between these pharmacokinetic properties and inhibition of platelet reactivity (p<0.01).

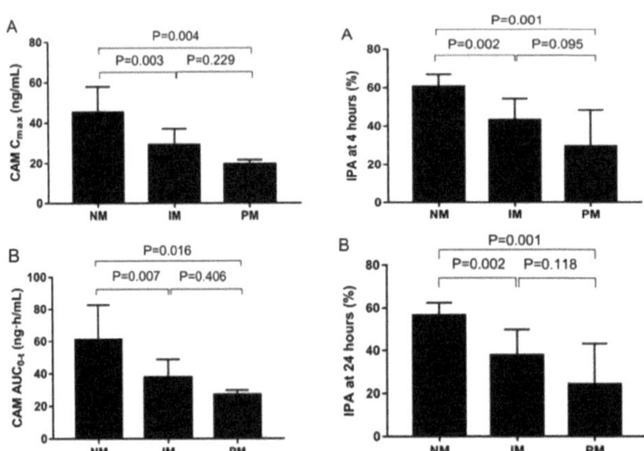

Figure 13: Impact of cytochrome P2C19*2 and cytochrome P2C19*3 polymorphisms on the pharmacokinetic properties of the active metabolite of clopidogrel and on the inhibition of platelet aggregation at 4h and 24h [97].

IPA: inhibition of platelet aggregation; CAM: active metabolite of clopidogrel; NM: normal metabolizers; IM: intermediate metabolizers; PM: poor metabolizers; LTA: light transmission aggregometry; AUC: area under curve; Cmax: maximum concentration.

A number of studies have also highlighted the clinical usefulness of genotyping patients taking clopidogrel. Furthermore, in 2010, the FDA (Food Drug Administration) issued a warning that clopidogrel may be less effective in patients carrying the LOF allele of CYP2C19*2 and that tests available to identify genetic differences in CYP2C19 function could be used**[98]**.

Some studies on the impact of CYP2C19 genetic polymorphisms and its associated genes on response to clopidogrel are summarised in **tableVI**.

Table VI: Consequences of genetic polymorphism of cytochrome P450 and its associated genes on the clinicobiological response to clopidogrel

Study	Method	Population	Number of patients	Polymorphism studied	Results
Angulo-Aguado et al.2021 [99]	PFA-200	SCA	166	CYP2C19 *2 CYP2C19 *17	The clopidogrel responder and non-responder groups showed no difference between the different genotypes. (p=0.21 for CYP2C19*2 and p=0.83 for the CYP2C19*17).
Aga 2020 [100]	VASP Index	Prophylaxis against cardiovascular disease	100	CYP2C19	The homozygous CYP2C19*1 allele was found to be the rapid metaboliser compared to the heterozygous CYP2C19*1 allele, whereas the CYP2C19*2 and CYP2C19*3 alleles were and were present in 28% of patients.
Yang et al. 2020 [101]	Verify Now® P2Y12	SCA	98	CYP2C19 *2 CYP2C19 *3 CYP2C19 *17	No association was observed between CYP2C19*3 and platelet reactivity on clopidogrel, but the frequency of HTPR (High on Treatment Platelet Reactivity) was significantly higher in patients carrying the CYP2C19*2 polymorphism in the homozygous state than in heterozygotes (p<0.05) and non-carriers (p<0.001). 100% of CYP2C19*2 carriers in the homozygous state maintained high platelet reactivity despite a dose of of clopidogrel.

Table VI (continued): Consequences of genetic polymorphism of cytochrome P450 and its associated genes on the clinicobiological response to clopidogrel

Study	Method	Population	Number of patients	Polymorphism studied	Results
Su et al. 2019 [102]	LTA	SCA	125	CYP2C19*3 CYP2C19*2	Carriage of the CYP2C19*2 mutated allele (OR=5.317; 95% CI [1.542-26.428]; p = 0.001) and CYP2C19*3 (OR= 4.295; IC95% [1.312-17.517]; p = 0.013) is one of the causes of CR in patients with ACS in china.
Chouchene et al. 2018 [96]	VerifyNow® P2Y12	SCA	150 : 76: diabetics 74: non-diabetics	CYP2C19*2	Carrying the CYP2C19*2 allele in diabetic patients was significantly associated with HTPR (p=0.032; OR= 4.437; 95% CI [1.134-17.359]). In contrast, in non-diabetic patients, there was no significant difference in platelet response to clopidogrel according to the presence or absence of a CYP2C19 * 2 allele (p = 0.759; OR= 1.260, IC 95% [0.288 - 5.522]).

ACS: acute coronary syndrome;LTA: Light Transmission Aggregometry; PFA: Platelet Function Analyzer;VASP: VASodilator Stimulated Phosphoprotein; HTPR: High on Treatment Platelet Reactivity;CR: Clopidogrel Resistance.

Alongside cytochrome CYP2C19, CYP3A4 is also involved in the formation of the active metabolite of clopidogrel and has several polymorphisms which may be responsible for the variability in platelet reactivity in patients treated with clopidogrel and may interfere with therapeutic response**[91]**. Mirzaev et al**[103]** concluded that there is no relationship between CYP3A4 activity and platelet reactivity on clopidogrel and that genotyping does not predict the antiplatelet effect of clopidogrel. Other studies have reported that of the CYP3A4 polymorphisms studied (CYP3A4*1B, CYP3A4*3, IVS7+258A>G, IVS7+894C>T, and IVS10+12G>A), only the IVS10+ 12G>A polymorphism in CYP3A4 had an impact on platelet aggregation in patients treated with clopidogrel, which may contribute to variability in response. However, further studies are needed to establish the clinical relevance of these polymorphisms.

CYP2C9*2 and *3 alleles may also contribute to the altered platelet response. Carriers of these variants have shown significant residual platelet reactivity under clopidogrel. In addition, these alleles influence the pharmacokinetic properties of the active metabolite**[104]**.

❖ **Carboxylesterase 1 gene polymorphism**

The vast majority of absorbed clopidogrel is diverted by CES1 into inactive carboxylic metabolites. Therefore, genetic variations affecting CES1 expression or activity are thought to be important determinants of response to clopidogrel.CES1 has two isotypes, CES1A1 (often referred to as CES1) and CES1P1. Previous studies have identified several SNPs in the coding region of CES1, including rs71647871 (G143E), rs71647872 (D260fs), and the intronic variant rs8192950**[91]**.

The G143E mutation reduces the catalytic activity of CES1. Lewis et al. found that carriers of the CES1 143E allele had higher levels of the active metabolite of clopidogrel and a better response to clopidogrel than carriers of the 143G allele (wild type) in healthy individuals. At the same time, in patients with coronary heart disease treated with In clopidogrel, the 143E allele reduced ADP-induced platelet aggregation and the risk of cardiovascular events. Tarkiainen et al. also reported in healthy volunteers that carriers of the CES1 143E allele have a greater AUC of clopidogrel and the active metabolite and lower P2Y12-mediated platelet aggregation. In addition, CES1P1 rs3785161 was found to be associated with an attenuated antiplatelet effect of clopidogrel in 162 patients with coronary heart disease**[105]**. Another unique study by Neuvonen et al**[106]** found that variants of the rs12443580 and rs8192935 polymorphisms of the CES1 gene had a significant effect on CES1 expression in whole blood, but not in liver, indicating the tissue-specific effect of these polymorphisms on CES1 expression.These polymorphisms did not affect clopidogrel pharmacokinetics; in comparison, the CES1c.428G>A allele was associated with a significant decrease in clopidogrel hydrolysis. Mirzaev et al**[107]** studied the effect of the rs2244613 polymorphism in the CES1 gene on antiplatelet treatment with clopidogrel. It was determined that a modification of CES1 at position c.1168-33A>C may hypothetically affect protein phosphorylation and influence the catalytic function of CES1.This polymorphism may modify the secondary structure of the CES1 protein and affect the interaction between the CES1 protein and the ligand**[107]**.

❖ **Genetic polymorphism affecting platelet P2Y12 receptors** P2Y12 is a platelet ADP receptor that plays an essential role i n platelet activation. The P2Y12 gene is located o n chromosome 3q24-q25. It spans 47 kb and consists of three exons and two introns. Polymorphism of the P2Y12 receptor has been shown to be an important determinant of the large inter-individual variability in platelet reactivity**[108]**.

Initially, five polymorphisms of the P2Y12 receptor gene were identified (**Figure 14**)**[109]**, four of which (i-C139T, iT744C, i-ins801A, G52T) were found to be in complete binding disequilibrium. They were designated as H1 and H2 haplotypes, with frequencies of 86% and 14% respectively.

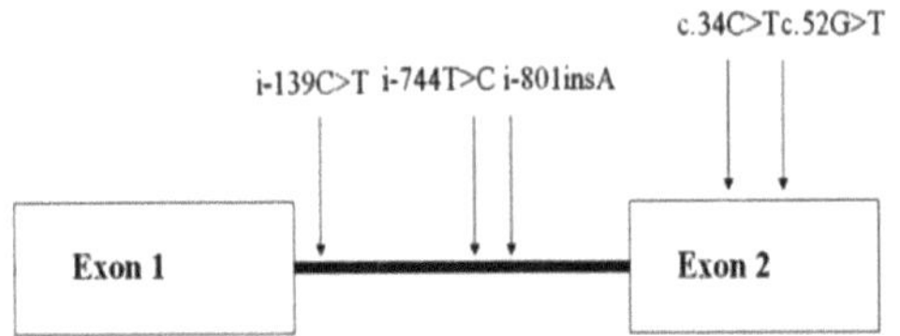

Figure 14: Schematic diagram of the locations of polymorphisms assessed in the P2Y12 gene [109].

Fontana et al**[110]** have shown that mutants homozygous for the H2 haplotype (744 T>C or 52G>T) of the P2Y12 gene are resistant to clopidogrel. They represent around 3% of the general population. They reported that ADP-induced platelet aggregation was associated with a P2Y12 H2 haplotype in healthy subjects. Staritz et al. contributed by reporting that a homozygous H2 genotype contributes to CR. Zoheir and colleagues showed an association between the rs2046934 T>C gene in P2Y12 and increased platelet activation in response to ADP**[111]**.

Li et al**[112]**showed that the rs6785930 C>T and rs6809699 G>T P2Y12 polymorphisms were associated with an increased risk of CR and subsequent cardiovascular events in Chinese patients with ACS after PCI. IL reported that carriers of the rs2046934 A allele (rs2046934 T>C) of P2Y12 had adverse events regardless of stent status (extracranial or intracranial). On the other hand, in a study by Nie et al**[113]**, the authors found a possible association between common genetic variations in P2Y12 and residual platelet reactivity to clopidogrel using thromboelastography in a Chinese ACS population after adjusting for the influence of CYP2C19*2 and *3 alleles. They selected the P2Y12 SNPs (rs6798347, rs6787801, rs6801273, rs6785930, and rs2046934) contained in the study.in the promoter region of the P2Y12 gene, which may modify its transcriptional activity rather than modifying the structure of the P2Y12 receptor. Their results show that the P2Y12 rs2046934 (T744C) allele was not significantly associated with High on Treatment Platelet Reactivity (HTPR).A 2019 meta-analysis by Zhao et al**[114]** of P2Y12 polymorphisms in patients treated with clopidogrel showed that ischaemic events are more frequent in patients with TT + TC vs CC genotypes of the P2Y12 C34T polymorphism. They showed that this polymorphism predicts the risk of recurrent adverse events, and that carriers of the T allele have a higher risk of ischaemic events despite taking clopidogrel. On the other hand, other studies have shown divergent results. According to a study by Ulehlova et al**[115]**, there was no statistically significant association between the C34T variant of the P2Y12 receptor and response to antiplatelet treatment with 75 mg clopidogrel.Siasos et al.**[116]** also showed that PRU assessed by VerifyNow did not differ between carriers and non-carriers of the C34T allele ($p = 0.41$) and that the C34T polymorphism had no impact on cardiovascular complications ($p = 0.17$).

3.1.2.8. Epigenetic factors predisposing to non-response to clopidogrel

Epigenetic alterations are mainly composed of non-coding RNAs, histone modification and DNA methylation. DNA methylation could have a significant influence on the response to clopidogrel. Studies suggest that DNA methylation modification, which occurs at cytosine phosphate-guanine (CpG) dinuclei, is a reliable and stable epigenetic modification and can actively remodel disease processes. Typically, CpG island hypermethylation (CGI) can induce silent transcriptase and influence the expression of targeted proteins. One study revealed that aberrant DNA methylation could participate à the onset and the development of plaques Several studies have attempted to determine the relationship between DNA methylation of other genes and CR. These genes were ABCB1, P2Y12 and PON1. Unlike CYP2C19, the CGI islands of these genes are located in the promoter region. DNA methylation in the promoter region inhibits transcription factor binding, thereby silencing gene expression. The P2Y12 study reported a lower percentage of DNA methylation in the clopidogrel-resistant group, but the PON1 study gave the opposite result. A lower percentage of P2Y12 methylation increases transcription of the gene and, as a result, more P2Y12 receptors are available for ADP binding, leading to increased platelet activity. The PON1 gene plays a role in the biotransformation of clopidogrel. Consequently, a higher percentage of methylation reduces transcription of the corresponding gene, leading to a reduction in the active metabolite of clopidogrel. In contrast, no significant relationship was found between DNA methylation of the ABCB1 gene and CR **[118]**. miRNAs are small, short, single-stranded non-coding RNAs, ~22 nucleotides in length. They can reduce mRNA expression by binding directly to the target mRNA and interfering with protein translation. Numerous studies have explored the link between specific mRNAs and miRNAs and platelet reactivity and activation. For example, studies have shown that miR-96 regulates the expression of platelet vesicle-associated microtubule protein 8, a critical component of platelet granule exocytosis. Others have also indicated that miR- 28 directly regulates the expression of the thrombopoietin receptor**[119]**. Of the 377 miRNAs observed in human platelets, miR-223 was the most differentially expressed in platelet-rich plasma compared with platelet-poor plasma and serum.Circulating platelet miRNAs are also thought to serve as indicators for tailoring anti-platelet therapies.The decrease in miR-223 expression in platelets and plasma predicted elevated platelet reactivity in patients treated with clopidogrel, indicating that the level of miR-223 could serve as a potential biomarker for predicting response to clopidogrel. MiR-26a has been shown to be involved in the regulation of platelet reactivity by clopidogrel via the regulation of vasodilator-stimulated phosphoprotein expression**[120]**.

3.1.3. Prasugrel

3.1.3.1. General

Formulated as a racemic hydrochloride salt, prasugrel [5-[(1RS)-2-cyclopropyl-1-(2-fluorophenyl)-2-oxoethyl]-4,5,6,7-tetrahydrothieno[3,2-c]pyridin-2-yl acetate hydrochloride(**figure15**), has the empirical formula C20H20FNO3S-HCl and a molecular weight of 409.9**[121]**.

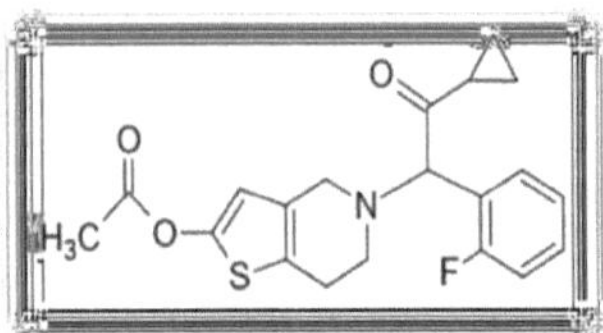

Figure 15: Chemical structure of prasugrel [121].

3.1.3.2. Pharmacodynamics

Like other thienopyridine derivatives, the active metabolite of prasugrel (R-138727) binds irreversibly to the P2Y12 receptor by forming disulphide bridges between extracellular cysteine residues at positions Cys17 and Cys270 to prevent platelet activation. In patients with stable coronary artery disease, prasugrel produces faster and more effective inhibition of platelet function than clopidogrel**[122]**. Its use in combination with aspirin is indicated as 1st line treatment (compared with the combination of aspirin and clopidogrel) in patients with ACS, with a view to coronary angioplasty**[122]**.

3.1.3.3. Pharmacokinetics

The parmacokinetic characteristics of prasugrel are summarised in the table VII.

Table VII: Pharmacokinetic characteristics of prasugrel [79].

Absorption	Elimination	Duration of effect
Per os Bioavailability ≈ 100%.	The prodrug is rapidly hydrolysed in the gut to thiolactone, which is then converted to an active metabolite in a single step, mainly by the enzymes CYP3A4 and CYP2B6. Its half-life elimination time is approximately 7 hours.	5 days

CYP3A4: cytochrome 3A4;CYP2B6: cytochrome 2B6

3.1.3.4. Sources of response variability

❖ **Non-genetic factors**

Several mechanisms may contribute to a poor response to prasugrel, making the treatment less effective (**table VIII**).

Table VIII:Effect of intrinsic factors on the pharmacokinetics and pharmacodynamics of prasugrel [79].

Intrinsic factors	Prasugrel
Low body weight	Increased exposure to active metabolites; Increased inhibition of platelet aggregation; risk of bleeding
Gender (women vs men)	Similar exposure in healthy subjects; Similar exposure in ACS patients; Similar PCI in healthy subjects; No PCI in ACS patients. clinically significant
Age	Similar exposure in healthy subjects and patients with stable coronary artery disease across the age range Similar PCI in healthy subjects across the age range Increase of exposure in ACS patients aged ≥ 75 years Clinically significant due to increased risk of bleeding
Renal insufficiency	Moderate: similar exposure and ICP; Severe: reduced exposure but similar ICP
Liver failure	Moderate: similar exposure and PCI; Severe: risk of bleeding increased; Clinically significant

ACS: acute coronary syndrome; PCI: percutaneous coronary intervention.

❖ Genetic factors

Several investigators have examined associations between CYP450 genotypes and response to prasugrel. One study reported an over-representation of the CYP2C9*2 variant in people with lower levels of platelet inhibition with prasugrel, while others found no significant effect of CYP2C9, CYP2C19, CYP2B6, CYP3A4 or CYP1A2 on prasugrel metabolite levels or antiplatelet effects**[123]**.

PEAR1 polymorphisms were studied for their variation in the effect of prasugrel. In a small study of 36 healthy native Chinese subjects, the effect of prasugrel was assessed by VerifyNow. The minor alleles of six SNPs (rs3737224, rs41273215, rs11264580, rs6671392, rs822441, and rs822442) were tested.polymorphisms have been associated with an increase in platelet reactivity to prasugrel. However, further study of these polymorphisms with prasugrel is needed to obtain tangible results**[43]**. Some studies on the impact of genetic polymorphisms on the response to prasugrel are summarised in **tableIX**.

Table IX: Variants influencing response to prasugrel [124].

References	Population	Gene	A variant	Remarks
Xiang et al. 2013	Volunteers in good health	PEAR1	rs822441	Patients with the CC genotype who are treated with prasugrel May have lowerlevels of platelet aggregation inhibition than patients with the CG or GG genotype.
Xiang et al. 2013	Volunteers in good health	PEAR1	rs12407843	AA genotype patients treated with prasugrel may have lower levels of platelet aggregation inhibition than AG or GG genotype patients.
Xiang et al. 2013	Volunteers in good health	PEAR1	rs77235035	AA genotype patients treated with prasugrel may have lower levels of inhibition of platelet aggregation than AA genotype patients treated with prasugrel. in patients with the AC or CC genotype.
Cuisset et al. 2012	ACS treated with PCI	CYP2C19	rs12248560	Patients with TT and CT genotype and coronary syndrome treated with prasugrel may have an increased risk of bleeding by compared with patients with the CC genotype.
Xiang et al. 2013	Volunteers in good health	PEAR1	rs3737224	Patients with the TT genotype treated with prasugrel may have lower levels of platelet aggregation inhibition compared to patients with the TT genotype. in patients with the CT or CC genotype.

Table IX (continued): Variants influencing response to prasugrel

References	Population	Gene	A variant	Remarks
Xiang et al. 2013	Volunteers in good health	PEAR1	rs822442	Patients with CC or AC genotype treated with prasugrel may have higher levels of platelet aggregation inhibition compared to AA genotype patients
Xiang et al. 2013	Volunteers in good health	PEAR1	rs41273215	Patients with TT genotype treated with prasugrel may have lower levels of platelet aggregation inhibition than patients with CT or CC genotype.
Cuisset et al. 2012; Brandt et al. 2007	ACS treated with PCI; healthy individuals	CYP2C19	rs4244285	GG genotype patients treated with prasugrel may have a lower rate of elevated platelet reactivity during treatment at 1 month compared to GG genotype patients. AG or AA. However, contradictory results have been reported.

ACS: acute coronary syndrome; PCI: Percutaneous Coronary Intervention.

3.2. Direct inhibitors

3.2.1. Ticagrélor

3.2.1.1. General

Ticagrelor was approved by the FDA in 2011 as the first direct inhibitor of the P2Y12 class. Its chemical structure, cyclopentyltriazolopyrimidine(**figure16**), gives it distinct pharmacokinetic and pharmacodynamic properties compared with clopidogrel and prasugrel. Unlike clopidogrel and prasugrel, ticagrelor acts as an ADP antagonist of the cyclopentyltriazolopyrimidine class.

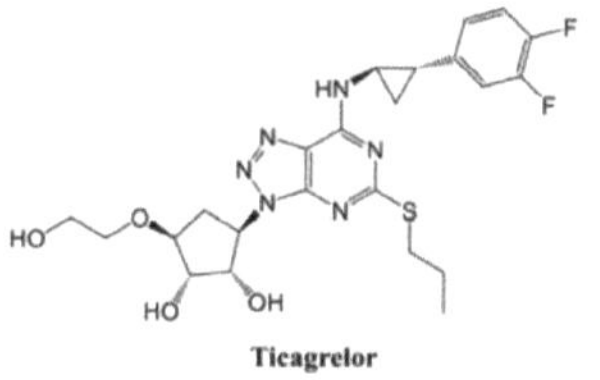

Figure 16: Chemical structure of ticagrelor [125].

3.2.1.2. Pharmacokinetics and pharmacodynamics

Ticagrelor binds reversibly to the P2Y12 receptor and inhibits platelet aggregation induced by ADP. It has a more rapid onset of action and more pronounced platelet inhibition than clopidogrel**[126]**.

Ticagrelor is absorbed orally and does not require metabolic activation to produce its clinical effect. It has an active metabolite, present in the blood at approximately one-third the concentration of the parent compound, as determined in phase I trials. After oral administration in healthy volunteers, the maximum effect on platelet inhibition was measured between 2 and 4 hours. The drug appears to have linear kinetics and, after twice-daily administration in patients with atherosclerotic disease, there is a linear, dose-dependent increase in ticagrelor and its active metabolite, with no age- or gender-related differences. The terminal half-life is approximately 7 hours**[127]**.

3.2.1.3. Variability in response to ticagrelor

Resistance to ticagrelor is less common than CR, but not uncommon. With the increasing applications of ticagrelor, some reports have recently emerged regarding ticagrelor resistance.Fluctuations in ticagrelor resistance rates can be attributed to differences in testing periods, methods used to define resistance, ethnicity of the population and sample size. Resistance to ticagrelor is mainly observed in elderly patients with co-morbidities such as diabetes and obesity**[128]**.

However, other genetic polymorphisms could have an influence on the pharmacodynamic or pharmacokinetic properties of this drug. Firstly, genetic polymorphisms in the ABCB1 (MDR1) gene may be a crucial factor. Numerous studies have observed associations between lower P-gp expression and SNPs 3435C > T, 1236C > T, 2677G > T/A, as well as 3435C > T. However, a randomised controlled trial found a different result, namely that ABCB1 genetic polymorphisms did not differ between ticagrelor-resistant and ticagrelor-sensitive patients **[129]**. Secondly, the role of the gut microbiome has been a hot topic in recent years, and studies have highlighted how the gut microbiota plays an important role in regulating P-gp expression. Metagenomic analysis of these core microbial communities revealed a positive correlation between specific short-chain fatty acids and the production of secondary bile acids such as lithocholic acid, deoxycholic acid and ursodeoxycholic acid, with P-gp expression**[130]**. These results suggest that elevated levels of these metabolites from the gut microbiome may be associated with increased P-gp expression, which in turn mediates ticagrelor efflux transport and leads to ticagrelor resistance. Results of a genome-wide association study revealed that the

SLCO1B1, CYP3A4 and UGT2B7 loci may be the most important for ticagrelor.rs62471956 and rs56324128 variants in the CYP3A4 gene were shown to influence ticagrelor metabolism, resulting in higher concentrations of the active metabolite. In addition, a variant rs113681054 in the SLCO1B1 gene influenced the concentrations of ticagrelor and its active metabolite, while the variant rs61361928 in the UGT2B7 gene was associated with higher concentrations of the active metabolite. However, most of these alleles were of minor frequency (<5%) and their impact was limited. Similar results were reported in a study published by Li et al. None of the polymorphisms studied (SLCO1B1 rs113681054, SLCO1B1*5, CYP3A4*1G and CYP3A5*3) had any effect on the pharmacokinetics or pharmacodynamics of ticagrelor **[131]**.

Although there is not yet sufficient evidence to determine whether these epigenetic factors affecting P2Y12 have a direct impact on the antiplatelet effects of ticagrelor, some studies have indicated that there is an association between specific miRNAs and platelet reactivity following treatment with ticagrelor. In patients treated with dual anti-platelet therapy with ticagrelor and aspirin, some authors observed that the increase in plasma miR-223 was significantly correlated with a decrease in platelet reactivity induced by ADP. In addition, other studies found that expression levels of miRNA 365-3p correlated with HTPR after treatment with ticagrelor. These results indicate the possibility of using specific miRNAs as biomarkers of ticagrelor resistance in the future**[132]**. Although the incidence of ticagrelor resistance is lower than that of clopidogrel, once resistance occurs, management will be difficult due to the paucity of effective alternative drugs. Therefore, how to detect and treat ticagrelor resistance is an important topic that needs to be explored further. resistance to ticagrelor are currently being studied (**figure17**). The form of ticagrelor may be an important factor influencing the absorption and bioavailability of ticagrelor. Thus, increasing its bioavailability by changing the form of ticagrelor may be a possible means of overcoming ticagrelor resistance **[133]**.

3.2.2. Cangrélor

Cangrélor binds directly to the P2Y12 receptor and therefore requires no bioactivation.It has a short plasma half-life of 3-5 minutes as it is rapidly inactivated by dephosphorylation by nucleotidases in the blood.Cangrélor metabolism is independent of hepatic CYP enzymes. Distribution was described by a two-compartment model and pharmacokinetics were dose-dependent up to the maximum dose tested of 4 µg/kg/min.Cangrélor binds reversibly to the P2Y12 receptor and has an extremely rapid onset and termination of action.

When administered as an intravenous bolus (15-30 μg/kg), followed by a continuous infusion (2-4 μg/kg/min), almost complete platelet inhibition is achieved in less than 2 minutes and platelet activity returns to baseline within 60-90 minutes of the end of the infusion**[79]**.

The impact of genetic polymorphisms in CYP enzymes on the pharmacokinetics or pharmacodynamics of cangrélor has not been studied because its metabolism is independent of CYP enzymes**[79]**.

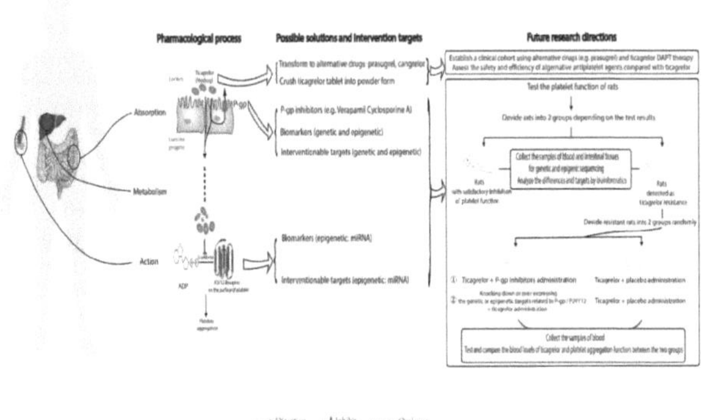

Figure 17:Possible targets for intervention and future directions for ticagrclor resistance research [128].

P-gp: P-glycoprotein; miRNA: microRNA

4. OTHER ANTIPLATELET AGENTS

4.1. Phosphodiesterase inhibitors

4.1.1. Dipyridamole

More than 50 years ago, dipyridamole (2,6-bis(diethanolamino)-4,8-dipiperidinopyrimido[5,4-d]pyrimidine) was synthesised and its initial use focused on its coronary vasodilator properties (**Figure 18**).

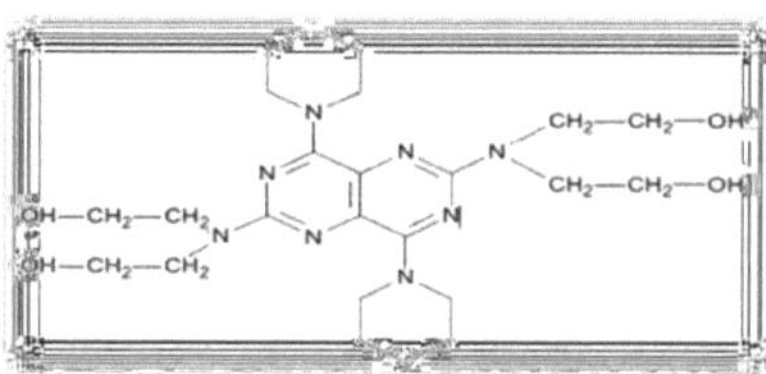

Figure 18: Chemical structure of dipyridamole [134].

By inhibiting phosphodiesterase, dipyridamole blocks the degradation of cAMP. Increased levels of cAMP reduce intracellular calcium and inhibit platelet activation. Dipyridamole also blocks the uptake of adenosine by platelets and other cells. This results in a further increase in local cAMP levels as the platelet adenosine A2 receptor is coupled to adenylate cyclase.Although there is variation in response to this product in terms of plasma concentration, to our knowledge there have been no resistance studies with this drug**[135]**.

4.1.2. Cilostazol

4.1.2.1. Molecule and Structure

Cilostazol is derived from 2-oxo-quinoline (6-[4-(1-cyclohexyl-1H-tetrazol-5-yl)butoxy]-3,4-dihydro-2(1H)-quinolinone) (**figure 19**). It was initially approved in Japan and other Asian countries in 1988 for the treatment of intermittent claudication **[136]**.

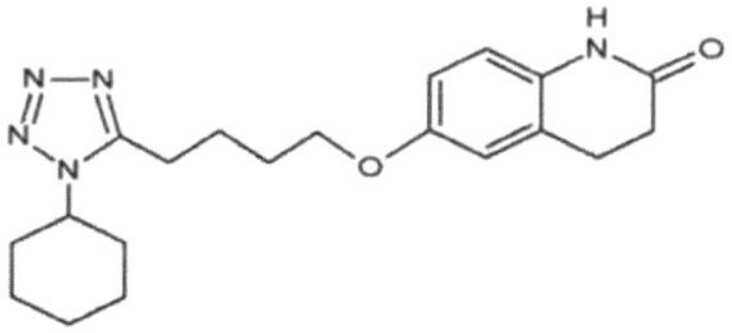

Figure 19: Chemical structure of cilostazol [136].

4.1.2.2. Mechanism of action

The pharmacology of cilostazol is multifaceted. It has a broad spectrum of pharmacological actions. Its main effect is the selective inhibition of type III cellular phosphodiesterase (PDE), which exists mainly in smooth muscle cells, myocytes, adipose tissue and cells of the digestive tract. Cilostazol therefore reversibly inhibits platelet aggregation induced by stimuli such as thrombin, ADP, collagen, AA, epinephrine and shear stress**[137]**.

4.1.2.3. Pharmacokinetics

Cilostazol is absorbed after oral administration, with peak plasma concentrations reached in 2 to 4 hours. The active form of cilostazol is 3,4-dehydro-cilostazol, which is 15 times more potent than cilostazol and 3 times more potent than an adenosine reuptake inhibitor. Cilostazol is mainly metabolised by CYP3A4, CYP2D6 and CYP2C19 among the cytochrome P450 enzymes in the liver, and the metabolites are largely excreted in the urine. The pharmacokinetic site of cilostazol varies between individuals due to genetic polymorphism of cytochrome P450. After administration, cilostazol has a biological half-life of approximately 10 to 14 hours**[137]**.

4.1.2.4. Indications

The pharmacological activities of cilostazol include anti-platelet activity, activity on endothelial cells and vasodilator activity, antiproliferative activity, neuroprotective activity and lipid activity. Cilostazol and its metabolites have been shown to increase intracellular cAMP via inhibition of PDE3-mediated hydrolysis and, subsequently, the active form of PKA is increased**[138]**.

4.1.2.5. Variability in response to cilostazol

The pharmacokinetic parameters of cilostazol have shown considerable inter-individual variability. A common cause of individual variation in drug response may be genetic polymorphism of drug enzymes**[139]**.

Although the enzymatic function of CYP3A5 sometimes overlaps with that of CYP3A4 in terms of substrate specificity, CYP3A4 and CYP3A5 convert cilostazol into different metabolites, a quinone-hydroxylated intermediate metabolite (OPC-13326) and a hexane-hydroxylated intermediate metabolite (OPC-13217), which are further metabolised to dehydrocilostazol (OPC-13015) and monohydroxycilostazol (OPC-13213), respectively.The CYP3A5*3 genotype is frequently observed in Japanese and Caucasian populations.

Homozygous carriers of the CYP3A5*3 genes lack functional CYP3A5 activity. One study showed that homozygous carriers of the CYP3A5*3 gene had slightly lower concentration/dose ratios of OPC-13213 and significantly higher plasma OPC13015 to cilostazol concentration levels than *1 carriers, in patients with cerebral infarction**[140]**.
However, in one study, CYP2C19 genotypes, but not CYP3A5 genotypes, affected the pharmacokinetics of cilostazol metabolites after a single administration in healthy volunteers. They hypothesised that the lack of genetic effect of CYP2C19 polymorphism on cilostazol pharmacokinetics is due to coadministration with CYP2C19 inhibitors**[141]**.

Other studies reported that no difference was observed in the AUC of cilostazol and OPC-13015 time-dependent concentration in healthy subjects after co-administration of clopidogrel between CYP2C19 genotype groups, whereas CYP3A5 genotypes affected the parameters. When CYP2C19 inhibitors are used concomitantly, CYP3A5 may play a more critical role in the metabolism of cilostazol, resulting in a greater influence of CYP3A5 polymorphisms on the pharmacokinetics of cilostazol. Another reason why CYP3A5 polymorphisms affected cilostazol metabolism more strongly than CYP2C19 may be the higher enzymatic affinity of CYP3A5 compared with CYP2C19 in the metabolism of cilostazol to OPC-13217 - an intermittent metabolite before OPC-13213 according to an in vitro study**[141]**.

4.2. Glycoprotein IIb IIIa inhibitors

4. 2.1. Overview of glycoprotein IIb IIIa inhibitors

GPIIb/IIIa inhibitors inhibit the interaction of the arginine, glycine and aspartic acid residues at position γ400-411 of fibrinogen with its platelet receptor, GP IIb/IIIa, expressed on activated platelets. Aggregation is therefore inhibited whatever the activator. Three compounds are currently available: abciximab, tirofiban and eptifibatide (**tableX**).

Table X:Pharmacology of glycoprotein IIb/IIIa inhibitors [142].

Features		GPIIb/IIIa inhibitors	
Generic name	Abciximab	Eptifibatide	Tirofiban
Description	Chimeric monoclonal antibody humanised mouse	Hepta-cyclic peptide	Nonpeptide
Route of administration	IV or IC	IV	IV
Duration of antiplatelet effect	24-48 hours	4-6 hours	6-8 hours
GPIIb/IIIa selectivity	No	Yes	Yes
Plasma half-life Platelet	10 to 30 minutes 4hours	2-2.5 hours	2 hours
Elimination	Reticuloendothelial system	Renal	Renal
Dose adjustment	Liver failure Elderly patients	Dialysis is a contraindication to the use of this drug, and it is imperative to adjust the dosage in patients with creatinine clearance of less than 50 mL/min.	Particular caution should be exercised in patients undergoing dialysis, and the dosage should be adjusted in patients with creatinine clearance of below 60 ml/min.
Indications	Prevention of ischemic cardiac complications in patients with ACS who are subjected to a PCI.	Patients with non-ST-segment elevation ACS undergoing PCI.	Patients with unstable angina or non-ST-segment elevation ACS undergoing PCI.

IC: intracardiac; IV: intravenous; ACS: acute coronary syndrome; PCI: percutaneous coronary intervention

4.2.2. Variability in response to glycoprotein IIb IIIa inhibitors

The fibrinogen receptor is the most abundant integrin on the platelet surface and consists of two subunits: glycoprotein IIb (GPIIb, integrin αIIb) and glycoprotein IIIa (GPIIIa, integrin β3). The GPIIIa subunit is polymorphic with single amino acid substitutions giving rise to a number of stable allelic variants.The PlA1/A2 diallel antigenic system is one of the most studied due to its involvement in alloimmunity and is the subject of ongoing controversy regarding its possible association with cardiovascular disease and resistance to antiplatelet agents.The presence of a proline residue at position 33 of the b3 subunit of abciximab may potentially have an impact on the efficacy of these drugs. One study examined the association between PLA1/PLA2 polymorphism and the in vitro efficacy of abciximab in patients undergoing percutaneous coronary angioplasty. Compared with PLA1/PLA1 homozygotes (n=66), PLA1/PLA2 heterozygotes (n=21) showed less inhibition of platelet aggregation t o ADP in the presence of abciximab, while the affinity of the molecule for the receptor did not appear to differ**[143]**.

These results are consistent with another study investigating the efficacy of eptifibatide in 23 individuals carrying the PLA2 polymorphism and 24 individuals carrying the PLA1/PLA1 polymorphism. The results of this study showed that eptifibatide was less effective in inhibiting platelet aggregation induced by ADP and collagen in PLA2 polymorphism carriers. Clinically, the association between the PLA1/PLA2 polymorphism and cardiovascular events in patients receiving anti-GPIIbIIIa treatment was studied in a subgroup of the OPUS-TIMI-16 study, a phase III trial evaluating the efficacy of an oral GPIIbIIIa antagonist (orbofiban)**[144]**.

Of the 10,288 ACS patients, genotyping was performed in 1,014 individuals. Overall, orbofiban did not demonstrate a reduction in cardiovascular events compared with placebo, but rather a In patients undergoing treatment, PLA2 polymorphism carriers (n = 170) had an increased risk of MI compared with PLA1/PLA1 carriers (n = 491, RR = 4.27, $p < 0.001$). Furthermore, while the risk of haemorrhage increased in a dose-dependent manner in PLA1/PLA1 carriers, PLA2 carriers did not have an increased risk of haemorrhage on treatment. The increase in cardiovascular events in patients treated with orbofiban may seem paradoxical, but some studies have revealed a prothrombotic effect of GPIIbIIIa antagonists, particularly when these drugs are administered at sub-therapeutic doses, by inducing a paradoxical activation of platelets and promoting an inflammatory response. It is therefore conceivable that the PLA1/PLA2 polymorphism may modulate this effect in certain circumstances**[135]**.

4.3. Protease-activated receptor inhibitors

4.3.1. Molecule and structure

Vorapaxar is a first-in-class Protease Activated Receptor1 (PAR1) inhibitor developed by Merck and Co for the secondary prevention of arterial thrombosis (**Figure 20**).

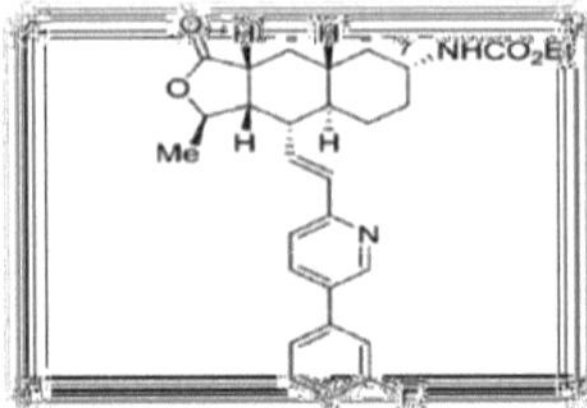

Figure 20: Chemical structure of vorapaxar [145].

4.3.2. Mechanism of action

Vorapaxar targets PAR1, the site of thrombin action. As an oral antagonist, vorapaxar is potent, selective and competitive against platelet PAR1, enabling it to inhibit the action of thrombin by reversible activation of this receptor. However, because of its long half-life (8 to 12 days), vorapaxar also exhibits characteristics of irreversible PAR1 inhibition. In parallel, atopaxar is another potent and selective PAR1 antagonist, offering an alternative option for modulating this signalling pathway**[31]**.

4.3.3. Pharmacokinetics

Vorapaxar is eliminated by metabolism, mainly catalysed by cytochrome P450 enzymes, in particular CYP3A4 and CYP2J2. The main route of elimination is faecal (58% of the administered dose), followed by urinary excretion (25%).vorapaxar pharmacokinetics are dose-dependent and steady state is reached within 21 days of daily administration with a 5- to 6-fold accumulation. Vorapaxar exhibits a multi-exponential disposition, with an effective half-life of 3 to 4 days and an apparent terminal elimination half-life of 8 days. The mean absolute bioavailability of vorapaxar is 100%. TheCmax of vorapaxar is reached 1 hour after administration of a single dose of 2.5 mg on an empty stomach**[146]**. Compared with vorapaxar, atopaxar has a slower onset of action (3.5 h) and its effect is more rapidly reversible (half-life of 23 h)**[146]**.

4.3.4. Variability in response to protease-activated receptor inhibitors

A limited number of polymorphisms in the PAR1 receptor gene have been reported in clinical studies.rs168753 intronic variation is associated with a reduction in PAR-1 receptors on the platelet surface and with response to agonist stimulation; the rs11267092 insertion/deletion variant has been evaluated for its protective role in venous thromboembolism. However, none of these variants has been associated with the clinical efficacy of the PAR1 antagonist vorapaxar or atopaxar**[147]**.

However, in a clinical study of 660 PCI patients, there was no evidence of increased MACEs or bleeding risk correlated with the polymorphism.The heritable interindividual variation in platelet reactivity was directly linked to PAR4. Platelet RNA and eXpression 1 (PRAX1) was designed to examine mRNAs and microRNAs associated with this difference in 154 healthy individuals who identified themselves as black or white. In this population, Edelstein et al.showed that black individuals had an increased platelet response to PAR4 stimulation, higher expression of phosphatidylcholine transfer protein and lower levels of miR-376c.The reverse was observed in white individuals.One study identified two additional polymorphisms that alter amino acids in PAR4 at positions 120 (Ala/Thr) and 296 (Phe/Val). The polymorphism at position 120 is common and is distributed by race.PAR4-120A has a lower reactivity and was found in 81% of white individuals compared with 37% of black individuals. In contrast, PAR4-120T was hyperreactive to agonists, resistant to a PAR4 antagonist and present in 63% of blacks compared with 19% of whites**[148]**.

5. DOES MODIFYING ANTI-PLATELET THERAPY ACCORDING TO THE RESULTS OF A GENETIC TEST CHANGE THE RESULTS?

The clinical utility of pharmacogenetic testing can be established if prospective data demonstrate that modification of antiplatelet therapy on the basis of pharmacogenetic testing can lead to a change in clinical outcomes. Several prospective studies and large meta-analyses primarily support the use of CYP2C19 pharmacogenetic testing in clinical practice. A prospective study of 1815 patients with stable coronary artery disease or ACS after PCI, in which genotyping results were available and the decision to choose a P2Y12 inhibitor was left to the physician, demonstrated that patients with CYP2C19 LOF alleles receiving ticagrelor or prasugrel rather than clopidogrel had significantly reduced MACEs.The lack of randomisation with assigned therapy may have biased the results, although propensity matching was performed to adjust for differences between groups. This study demonstrated the beneficial effect on actual clinical outcomes of providing CYP2C19 pharmacogenetic test results to the medical practitioner **[149]**.A recent meta-analysis including 15,949 patients (77% PCI, 98% ACS) from 7 randomised controlled trials reported that treatment with prasugrel or ticagrelor reduced major ischaemic events compared with clopidogrel in CYP2C19 LOF carriers, whereas no difference was observed in non-carriers. The results showed a marked interaction between genotype and treatment ($p = 0.013$), leading to the conclusion that the benefit of prasugrel or ticagrelor compared with clopidogrel was mainly due to CYP2C19 genotype status**[150]**. This study therefore lays the foundations for a pharmacogenetic test of CYP2C19 to identify and treat LOF carriers with ticagrelor or prasugrel and non-carriers with clopidogrel (**figure21**). In addition, another meta-analysis involving 20,743 patients, including 11 randomised controlled trials and 3 observational studies, demonstrated that guided selection of antiplatelet therapy using CYP2C19 genetic testing and platelet function tests significantly improved the frequency of MACEs and reduced individual ischaemic outcomes, with a significant reduction in minor bleeding.

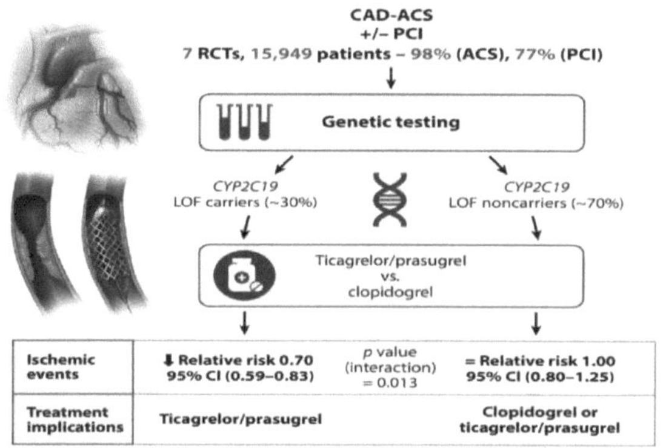

Figure 21: Proposed algorithm using CYP2C19 pharmacogenetic testing to individualise treatment with oral P2Y12 inhibitors in patients with coronary artery disease [149].

ACS:Acute coronary syndrome;CAD: Coronary artery disease; CI: Confidence interval; LOF: Loss-of-function; PCI: Percutaneous coronary intervention; RCT: Randomized clinical trial.

CONCLUSION

Antiplatelet therapies remain an essential tool for reducing the risk of developing clinically apparent atherothrombotic disease and are a mainstay of therapy for patients suffering from cardiovascular disease, cerebrovascular disease and peripheral arterial disease. Strategies to intensify antiplatelet therapy need to be complemented by approaches to target thrombosis while preserving haemostasis. A number of new anti-platelet therapies in development target a wide range of receptors and signalling pathways that have not been explored and offer enormous potential to improve patient outcomes by maintaining anti-platelet efficacy and preserving haemostasis. In recent years, improvements in medical practice and the development of antiplatelet response assessment have made it possible to better define therapeutic options in the case of a patient who is 'resistant' to antiplatelets, particularly in response to clopidogrel. Pharmacogenetics is increasingly recognised as a key element in the prescribing of pharmaceutical products, as more data becomes available. This is due to factors such as the increasing availability of genetic analyses and falling costs. This has stimulated the development of pharmacogenetic programmes at clinical sites in an attempt to integrate pharmacogenetics at a clinical level. When used for this purpose, the results of genetic tests can be used to identify the optimal drug class for each patient. In the case of antiplatelet drugs, due to the lack of randomised controlled data to support routine genetic testing, the AHA/ACC guidelines on the duration of antiplatelet agents have recommended against routine testing. Similarly, although the CPIC or FDA do not specifically advise routine genetic testing, it is advisable to select the optimal antiplatelet agent for the patient.patient if pharmacogenetic information is available. This is particularly true for CYP2C19 alleles with loss of function, where P2Y12 antagonists to clopidogrel (such as prasugrel or ticagrelor) are used. This approach to pharmacogenetics has been useful for classes of drugs whose traditional mechanism of action is well understood. Although this approach has been very successful in determining the prevalence of non-functional and increased function variants in these genes, it is quite slow and involves the analysis of genes that have a clear impact on the drug or its metabolism. Genome-wide association studies have been used at population level in other specialities to successfully assess genotypic variants that can predict response to treatment. This allows broader screening for genotypic variants associated with variations in plasma drug concentrations, for example.

REFERENCES

1. **Kang J, Park KW, Lee H, Hwang D, Yang HM, Rha SW, et al.** Aspirin versus clopidogrel for long-term maintenance monotherapy after percutaneous coronary intervention: The HOST-EXAM extended study. Circulation. 2023;147:108-17.

2. **Pultar J, Wadowski PP, Panzer S, Gremmel T.** Oral antiplatelet agents in cardiovascular disease. Vasa. 2019;48:291-302.

3. **Chang WC, Tanoshima R, Ross CJD, Carleton BC.** Challenges and opportunities in implementing pharmacogenetic testing in clinical settings. Annu Rev Pharmacol Toxicol. 2021;61:65-84.

4. **Koo SH, Lee EJ.** Pharmacogenetics approach to therapeutics. Clin Exp Pharmacol Physiol. 2006;33:525-32.

5. **Bourel M, Ardaillou R.** Pharmacogenetics and pharmacogenomics. Bull Acad Natl Med. 2006;190:9-23.

6. **Charlab R, Zhang L.** Pharmacogenomics: historical perspective and current status. Methods Mol Biol. 2013;1015:3-22.

7. **Van Driest SL, Cascorbi I.** Progress and challenges in pharmacogenomics. Clin Pharmacol Ther. 2021;110:529-32.

8. **Osanlou O, Pirmohamed M, Daly AK.** Pharmacogenetics of adverse drug reactions. Adv Pharmacol. 2018;83:155-90.

9. **Daali Y.** Personalized Medicine: Pharmacokinetics. J Pers Med. 2022;12:1660.

10. **Ahmed S, Zhou Z, Zhou J, Chen SQ.** Pharmacogenomics of drug metabolizing enzymes and transporters: relevance to precision medicine. Genomics Proteomics Bioinformatics. 2016;14:298-313.

11. **Jukic MM, Lauschke VM, Saito T, Hiratsuka M, Ingelman-Sundberg M.** Functional characterization of CYP2D7 gene variants. Pharmacogenomics. 2018;19:931-6.

12. **Taylor C, Crosby I, Yip V, Maguire P, Pirmohamed M, Turner RM.** A review of the important role of CYP2D6 in pharmacogenomics. Genes (Basel). 2020;11:1295.

13. **Richards-Belle A, Austin-Zimmerman I, Wang B, Zartaloudi E, Cotic M, Gracie C, et al.** Associations of antidepressants and antipsychotics with

lipid parameters: Do CYP2C19/CYP2D6 genes play a role? A UK population-based study. J Psychopharmacol. 2023;37:396-407.

14. **Dorji PW, Wangchuk S, Boonprasert K, Tarasuk M, Na-Bangchang K.** Pharmacogenetic relevant polymorphisms of CYP2C9, CYP2C19, CYP2D6, and CYP3A5 in Bhutanese population. Drug Metab Pers Ther. 2019;34(4):1-14.

15. **Miteva-Marcheva NN, Ivanov HY, Dimitrov DK, Stoyanova VK.** Application of pharmacogenetics in oncology. Biomark Res. 2020;8:32.

16. **Carranza-Leon D, Dickson AL, Gaedigk A, Stein CM, Chung CP.** CYP2D6 genotype and reduced codeine analgesic effect in real-world clinical practice. Pharmacogenomics J. 2021;21:484-90.

17. **Dietz N, Ruff C, Giugliano RP, Mercuri MF, Antman EM.** Pharmacogenetic-guided and clinical warfarin dosing algorithm assessments with bleeding outcomes risk-stratified by genetic and covariate subgroups. Int J Cardiol. 2020;317:159-66.

18. **Firasat S, Raza A, Khan AR, Abid A.** The prevalence of pharmacogenetic variants of vitamin K epoxide reductase complex subunit 1 gene (rs9923231), cytochrome P450 family 2 subfamily C member 9 gene (rs1799853) and cytochrome P450 family 3 subfamily-A member-5 gene (rs776746) among 13 ethnic groups of Pakistan. Mol Biol Rep. 2023;50:4017-27.

19. **Magavern EF, van Heel DA, Smedley D, Caulfield MJ.** CYP2C19 loss of function alleles are not associated with higher prevalence of gastrointestinal bleeds in those who have been prescribed antidepressants: Analysis in a British-South Asian cohort. Br J Clin Pharmacol. 2023;doi: 10.1111/bcp.15762 In press.

20. **Scheibner A, Remmel R, Schladt D, Oetting WS, Guan W, Wu B, et al.** Tacrolimus elimination in four patients with a CYP3A5*3/*3 CYP3A4*22/*22 genotype combination. Pharmacotherapy. 2018;38:e46-52.

21. **Tillman E, Nikirk MG, Chen J, Skaar TC, Shugg T, Maddatu JP, et al.** Implementation of clinical cytochrome P450 3A genotyping for tacrolimus dosing in a large kidney transplant program. J Clin Pharmacol. 2023;doi: 10.1002/jcph.2249 In press.

22. **Lefèvre F, Boutry M.** Towards identification of the substrates of ATP-binding cassette transporters. Plant Physiol. 2018;178:18-39.

23. **Campion DP, Dowell FJ.** Translating pharmacogenetics and pharmacogenomics to the clinic: progress in human and veterinary medicine. Front Vet Sci. 2019;6:22.

24. van Heteren DM, Lijfering WM, van der Meer FJM, Reitsma PH, Swen JJ, Bos MH, et al. Association of VKORC1 polymorphisms and major bleedings in patients who are treated with vitamin K antagonists. J Intern Med. 2023;293:124-7.

25. Sadee W, Wang D, Hartmann K, Toland AE. Pharmacogenomics: driving personalized medicine. Pharmacol Rev. 2023;75:789-814.

26. Haidar CE, Crews KR, Hoffman JM, Relling MV, Caudle KE. Advancing pharmacogenomics from single-gene to preemptive testing. Annu Rev Genomics Hum Genet. 2022;23:449-73.

27. Nicholson WT, Formea CM, Matey ET, Wright JA, Giri J, Moyer AM. Considerations when applying pharmacogenomics to your practice. Mayo Clin Proc. 2021;96:218-30.

28. Ho TT, Gift M, Alexander E. Prioritizing pharmacogenomics implementation initiates: a survey of healthcare professionals. Per Med. 2022;19:15-23.

29. Rezabakhsh A, Mahmoodpoor A, Soleimanpour H. Historical perspective of aspirin: A journey from discovery to clinical practice Ancient and modern history. J Cardiovasc Thorac Res. 2021;13:179-80.

30. Murtaza G, Karim S, Najam-ul-Haq M, Ahmad M, Ismail T, Khan SA, et al. Interaction analysis of aspirin with selective amino acids. Acta Pol Pharm. 2014;71:139-43.

31. Kolandaivelu K, Bhatt DL. Novel antiplatelet therapies. In: Michelson AD, editor. Platelets. 4th edition. Amsterdam: Elsevier; 2019.p.991 1015.

32. Atallah A, Lecarpentier E, Goffinet F, Gaucherand P, Doret-Dion M, Tsatsaris V. Aspirin and preeclampsia. Presse Med. 2019;48(1 Pt 1):34-45.

33. Patrono C. Aspirin. In: Michelson AD, editor. Platelets. 4th edition.

Amsterdam: Elsevier; 2019.p.921-36.

34. Tanasescu S, Lévesque H, Thuillez C. Pharmacology of aspirin. Rev Med Interne. 2000;21 Suppl 1:18s-26s.

35. Russo NW, Petrucci G, Rocca B. Aspirin, stroke and drug-drug interactions. Vascul Pharmacol. 2016;87:14-22.

36. Marquis-Gravel G, Roe MT, Harrington RA, Muñoz D, Hernandez AF, Jones WS. Revisiting the role of aspirin for the primary prevention of cardiovascular disease. Circulation. 2019;140:1115-24.

37. **Dimmitt SB, Floyd CN, Ferner RE.** Antithrombotic dose: Some observations from published clinical trials. Br J Clin Pharmacol. 2019;85:2194-7.

38. **Kalra K, Franzese CJ, Gesheff MG, Lev EI, Pandya S, Bliden KP, et al.** Pharmacology of antiplatelet agents. Curr Atheroscler Rep. 2013;15:371.

39. **Cai G, Zhou W, Lu Y, Chen P, Lu Z, Fu Y.** Aspirin resistance and other aspirin-related concerns. Neurol Sci. 2016;37:181-9.

40. **Van Oosterom N, Barras M, Cottrell N, Bird R.** Platelet function assays for the diagnosis of aspirin resistance. Platelets. 2022;33:329-38.

41. **Le Quellec S, Bordet JC, Negrier C, Dargaud Y.** Comparison of current platelet functional tests for the assessment of aspirin and clopidogrel response. A review of the literature. Thromb Haemost. 2016;116:638-50.

42. **Ferreira M, Freitas-Silva M, Assis J, Pinto R, Nunes JP, Medeiros R.** The emergent phenomenon of aspirin resistance: insights from genetic association studies. Pharmacogenomics. 2020;21:125-40.

43. **O'connor CT, Kiernan TJ, Yan BP.** The genetic basis of antiplatelet and anticoagulant therapy: A pharmacogenetic review of newer antiplatelets (clopidogrel, prasugrel and ticagrelor) and anticoagulants (dabigatran, rivaroxaban, apixaban and edoxaban). Expert Opin Drug Metab Toxicol. 2017;13:725-39.

44. **Halushka MK, Walker LP, Halushka PV.** Genetic variation in cyclooxygenase 1: effects on response to aspirin. Clin Pharmacol Ther. 2003;73:122-30.

45. **Lepäntalo A, Mikkelsson J, Reséndiz JC, Viiri L, Backman JT, Kankuri E, et al.** Polymorphisms of COX-1 and GPVI associate with the antiplatelet effect of aspirin in coronary artery disease patients. Thromb Haemost. 2006;95:253-9.

46. **Maree AO, Curtin RJ, Chubb A, Dolan C, Cox D, O'Brien J, et al.** Cyclooxygenase-1 haplotype modulates platelet response to aspirin. J Thromb Haemost. 2005;3:2340-5.

47. **Würtz M, Kristensen SD, Hvas AM, Grove EL.** Pharmacogenetics of the antiplatelet effect of aspirin. Curr Pharm Des. 2012;18:5294-308.

48. **Kirac D, Yaman AE, Doran T, Mihmanli M, Keles EC.** COX-1, COX-2 and CYP2C19 variations may be related to cardiovascular events due to acetylsalicylic acid resistance. Mol Biol Rep. 2022;49:3007-14.

49. **Chakroun T, Addad F, Yacoub S, Abderrezak F, Gerotziafas GT, Abdelkafi S, et al.** The cyclooxygenase-1 C50T polymorphism is not associated with aspirin responsiveness status in stable coronary artery disease in Tunisian patients. Genet Test Mol Biomarkers. 2011;15:513-6.

50. **Wang H, Sun X, Dong W, Cai X, Zhou Y, Zhang Y, et al.** Association of GPIa and COX-2 gene polymorphism with aspirin resistance. J Clin Lab Anal. 2018;32:e22331.

51. **Sharma V, Kaul S, Al-Hazzani A, Alshatwi AA, Jyothy A, Munshi A.** Association of COX-2 rs20417 with aspirin resistance. J Thromb Thrombolysis. 2013;35:95-9.

52. **Cipollone F, Toniato E, Martinotti S, Fazia M, Iezzi A, Cuccurullo C, et al.** A polymorphism in the cyclooxygenase 2 gene as an inherited protective factor against myocardial infarction and stroke. JAMA. 2004;291:2221-8.

53. **Szczeklik A, Undas A, Sanak M, Frolow M, Wegrzyn W.** Relationship between bleeding time, aspirin and the PlA1/A2 polymorphism of platelet glycoprotein IIIa. Br J Haematol. 2000;110:965-7.

54. **Wang J, Liu J, Zhou Y, Wang F, Xu K, Kong D, et al.** Association among PlA1/A2 gene polymorphism, laboratory aspirin resistance and clinical outcomes in patients with coronary artery disease: An updated meta-analysis. Sci Rep. 2019;9:13177.

55. **Silva GF da, Lopes BM, Moser V, Ferreira LE.** Impact of pharmacogenetics on aspirin resistance: a systematic review. Arq Neuropsiquiatr. 2023;81:62-73.

56. **Zhao Y, Yang S, Wu M.** Mechanism of improving aspirin resistance: blood-activating herbs combined with aspirin in treating atherosclerotic cardiovascular diseases. Front Pharmacol. 2021;12:794417.

57. **Paseban M, Marjaneh RM, Banach M, Riahi MM, Bo S, Sahebkar A.** Modulation of microRNAs by aspirin in cardiovascular disease. Trends Cardiovasc Med. 2020;30:249-54.

58. **Goodman T, Sharma P, Ferro A.** The genetics of aspirin resistance. Int J Clin Pract. 2007;61:826-34.

59. **Jefferson BK, Foster JH, McCarthy JJ, Ginsburg G, Parker A, Kottke-Marchant K, et al.** Aspirin resistance and a single gene. Am J Cardiol. 2005;95:805-8.

60. **Zhang S, Zhu J, Li H, Wang L, Niu J, Zhu B, et al.** Study of the association of PEAR1, P2Y12, and UGT2A1 polymorphisms with platelet

reactivity in response to dual antiplatelet therapy in Chinese patients. Cardiology. 2018;140:21-9.

61. **Zhao J, Chen F, Lu L, Tang H, Yang R, Wang Y, et al.** Effect of 106PEAR1 and 168PTGS1 genetic polymorphisms on recurrent ischemic stroke in Chinese patient. Medicine (Baltimore). 2019;98:e16457.

62. **Peng LL, Zhao YQ, Zhou ZY, Jin J, Zhao M, Chen XM, et al.** Associations of MDR1, TBXA2R, PLA2G7, and PEAR1 genetic polymorphisms with the platelet activity in Chinese ischemic stroke patients receiving aspirin therapy. Acta Pharmacol Sin. 2016;37:1442-8.

63. **Du G, Lin Q, Wang J.** A brief review on the mechanisms of aspirin resistance. Int J Cardiol. 2016;220:21-6.

64. **Xu K, Ye S, Zhang S, Yang M, Zhu T, Kong D, et al.** Impact of platelet endothelial aggregation receptor-1 genotypes on platelet reactivity and early cardiovascular outcomes in patients undergoing percutaneous coronary intervention and treated with aspirin and clopidogrel. Circ Cardiovasc Interv. 2019;12:e007019.

65. **Xue M, Yang X, Yang L, Kou N, Miao Y, Wang M, et al.** rs5911 and rs3842788 genetic polymorphism, blood stasis syndrome, and plasma TXB2 and hs-CRP levels are associated with aspirin resistance in Chinese chronic stable angina patients. Evid Based Complement Alternat Med. 2017;2017:9037094.

66. **Yi X, Cheng W, Lin J, Zhou Q, Wang C.** Interaction between COX-1 and COX-2 variants associated with aspirin resistance in chinese stroke patients. J Stroke Cerebrovasc Dis. 2016;25:2136-44.

67. **Abderrazek F, Chakroun T, Addad F, Dridi Z, Gerotziafas G, Gamra H, et al.** The GPIIIa PlA polymorphism and the platelet hyperactivity in Tunisian patients with stable coronary artery disease treated with aspirin. Thromb Res. 2010;125:e265-8.

68. **Singh S, de Ronde MWJ, Creemers EE, Van der Made I, Meijering R, Chan MY, et al.** Low miR-19b-1-5p expression is related to aspirin resistance and major adverse cardio- cerebrovascular events in patients with acute coronary syndrome. J Am Heart Assoc. 2021;10:e017120.

69. **Jing Y, Yue X, Yang S, Li S.** Association of aspirin resistance with increased mortality in ischemic stroke. J Nutr Health Aging. 2019;23:266-70.

70. **Wiśniewski A.** Multifactorial background for a low biological response to antiplatelet agents used in stroke prevention. Medicina (Kaunas). 2021;57:59.

71. **Khan H, Kanny O, Syed MH, Qadura M.** Aspirin resistance in vascular

disease: a review highlighting the critical need for improved point-of-care testing and personalized therapy. Int J Mol Sci. 2022;23:11317.

72. **Wang Y, Pan Y, Li H, Amarenco P, Denison H, Evans SR, et al.** Efficacy and safety of ticagrelor and aspirin in patients with moderate ischemic stroke: an exploratory analysis of the THALES randomized clinical trial. JAMA Neurol. 2021;78:1091-8.

73. **Bergmark BA, Bhatt DL, Steg PG, Budaj A, Storey RF, Gurmu Y, et al.** Long-term ticagrelor in patients with prior coronary stenting in the PEGASUS-TIMI 54 trial. J Am Heart Assoc. 2021;10:e020446.

74. **Cattaneo M.** P2Y12 Antagonists. In: Michelson AD, editor. Platelets. 4th edition. Amsterdam: Elsevier; 2019.p.937-56.

75. **Aoki M, Naya M, Arima S, Shinohara K, Kato M, Shibuya K, et al.** Mixture of clopidogrel bisulfate and magnesium oxide tablets reduces clopidogrel dose administered through a feeding tube. J Pharm Health Care Sci. 2021;7:18.

76. **Becker DE.** Antithrombotic drugs: pharmacology and implications for dental practice. Anesth Prog. 2013;60:72-80.

77. **Gaussem P, Ajzenberg N.** Antiplatelet therapies. EMC - AKOS (Traité de Médecine) 2014:1-9 [Article 4-0200].

78. **Angiolillo DJ, Fernandez-Ortiz A, Bernardo E, Alfonso F, Macaya C, Bass TA, et al.** Variability in individual responsiveness to clopidogrel: clinical implications, management, and future perspectives. J Am Coll Cardiol. 2007;49:1505-16.

79. **Schilling U, Dingemanse J, Ufer M.** Pharmacokinetics and pharmacodynamics of approved and investigational P2Y12 receptor antagonists. Clin Pharmacokinet. 2020;59:545-66.

80. **Perera KS, Pearce LA, Sharma M, Benavente O, Connolly SJ, Hart RG, et al.** Predictors of mortality in patients with atrial fibrillation (from the atrial fibrillation clopidogrel trial with irbesartan for prevention of vascular events [ACTIVE A]). Am J Cardiol. 2018;121:584-9.

81. **Guirgis M, Thompson P, Jansen S.** Review of aspirin and clopidogrel resistance in peripheral arterial disease. J Vasc Surg. 2017;66:1576-86.

82. **Gupta R, Kirtane AJ, Liu Y, Crowley A, Witzenbichler B, Rinaldi MJ, et al.** Impact of smoking on platelet reactivity and clinical outcomes after percutaneous coronary intervention: findings from the ADAPT-DES study. Circ

Cardiovasc Interv. 2019;12:e007982.

83. Amin AM, Sheau Chin L, Azri Mohamed Noor D, Sk Abdul Kader MA, Kah Hay Y, Ibrahim B. The personalization of clopidogrel antiplatelet therapy: the role of integrative pharmacogenetics and pharmacometabolomics. Cardiol Res Pract. 2017;2017:8062796.

84. Biswas M, Rahaman S, Biswas TK, Ibrahim B. Effects of the ABCB1 C3435T single nucleotide polymorphism on major adverse cardiovascular events in acute coronary syndrome or coronary artery disease patients undergoing percutaneous coronary intervention and treated with clopidogrel: A systematic review and meta-analysis. Expert Opin Drug Saf. 2020;19:1605-16.

85. Su J, Yu Q, Zhu H, Li X, Cui H, Du W, et al. The risk of clopidogrel resistance is associated with ABCB1 polymorphisms but not promoter methylation in a Chinese Han population. PLoS One. 2017;12:e0174511.

86. Li XQ, Ma N, Li XG, Wang B, Sun SS, Gao F, et al. Association of PON1, P2Y12 and COX1 with recurrent ischemic events in patients with extracranial or intracranial stenting. PLoS One. 2016;11:e0148891.

87. Zhai Y, He H, Ma X, Xie J, Meng T, Dong Y, et al. Meta-analysis of effects of ABCB1 polymorphisms on clopidogrel response among patients with coronary artery disease. Eur J Clin Pharmacol. 2017;73:843-54.

88. Pan Y, Elm JJ, Li H, Easton JD, Wang Y, Farrant M, et al. Outcomes Associated with clopidogrel-aspirin use in minor stroke or transient ischemic attack: a pooled analysis of clopidogrel in high-risk patients with acute non-disabling cerebrovascular events (CHANCE) and platelet- oriented inhibition in new TIA and minor ischemic stroke (POINT) trials. JAMA Neurol. 2019;76:1466-73.

89. Zhang XG, Zhu XQ, Xue J, Li ZZ, Jiang HY, Hu L, et al. Personalised antiplatelet therapy based on pharmacogenomics in acute ischaemic minor stroke and transient ischaemic attack: study protocol for a randomised controlled trial. BMJ Open. 2019;9:e028595.

90. Tanaka K, Matsumoto S, Ainiding G, Nakahara I, Nishi H, Hashimoto T, et al. PON1 Q192R is associated with high platelet reactivity with clopidogrel in patients undergoing elective neurointervention: A prospective single-center cohort study. PLoS One. 2021;16:e0254067.

91. Zhang YJ, Li MP, Tang J, Chen XP. Pharmacokinetic and pharmaco-dynamic responses to clopidogrel: evidences and perspectives. Int J Environ Res Public Health. 2017;14:301.

92. Pereira NL, Rihal CS, So DY, Rosenberg Y, Lennon RJ, Mathew V, et al. Clopidogrel pharmacogenetics. Circ Cardiovasc Interv. 2019;12:e007811.

93. Velazquez MN, Parween S, Udhane SS, Pandey AV. Variability in human drug metabolizing cytochrome P450 CYP2C9, CYP2C19 and CYP3A5 activities caused by genetic variations in cytochrome P450 oxidoreductase. Biochem Biophys Res Commun. 2019;515:133-8.

94. Akkaif MA, Daud NA, Sha'aban A, Ng ML, Abdul Kader MA, Noor DA, et al. The role of genetic polymorphism and other factors on clopidogrel resistance (CR) in an Asian population with coronary heart disease (CHD). Molecules. 2021;26:1987.

95. Thomas CD, Williams AK, Lee CR, Cavallari LH. Pharmacogenetics of P2Y12 receptor inhibitors. Pharmacotherapy. 2023;43:158-75.

96. Chouchene S, Dabboubi R, Raddaoui H, Abroug H, Hamda KB, Fredj SH, et al. Clopidogrel utilization in patients with coronary artery disease and diabetes mellitus: should we determine CYP2C192 genotype? Eur J Clin Pharmacol. 2018;74:1567-74.

97. Song BL, Wan M, Tang D, Sun C, Zhu YB, Linda N, et al. Effects of CYP2C19 genetic polymorphisms on the pharmacokinetic and pharmacodynamic properties of clopidogrel and its active metabolite in healthy Chinese subjects. Clin Ther. 2018;40:1170-8.

98. Li X, Wang Z, Wang Q, Xu Q, Lv Q. Clopidogrel-associated genetic variants on inhibition of platelet activity and clinical outcome for acute coronary syndrome patients. Basic Clin Pharmacol Toxicol. 2019;124:84-93.

99. Angulo-Aguado M, Panche K, Tamayo-Agudelo CA, Ruiz-Torres DA, Sambracos-Parrado S, Niño-Orrego MJ, et al. A pharmacogenetic study of CYP2C19 in acute coronary syndrome patients of Colombian origin reveals new polymorphisms potentially related to clopidogrel therapy. J Pers Med. 2021;11:400.

100. Aga QA, Hasan MK, Nassir KF, Aga LA, Al-Jaidi BA, Aldhoun M, et al. Prevalence and types of genetic polymorphisms of CYP2C19 and their effects on platelet aggregation inhibition by clopidogrel. Eur Rev Med Pharmacol Sci. 2020;24:11286-94.

101. Yang Y, Zhang W, Li P, Gu Y, Ma L, Fan M. Association of CYP2C19

2 polymorphisms and high on-treatment platelet reactivity in acute myocardial infarction or coronary artery in-stent restenosis patients during dual antiplatelet therapy. Med Drug Discov. 2020;6:100038.

102. Su Q, Li J, Tang Z, Yang S, Xing G, Liu T, et al. Association of CYP2C19 polymorphism with clopidogrel resistance in patients with acute coronary syndrome in China. Med Sci Monit. 2019;25:7138-48.

103. Mirzaev KB, Samsonova KI, Potapov PP, Andreev DA, Grishina EA, Ryzhikova KA, et al. Genotyping and phenotyping CYP3A4\CYP3A5: no association with antiplatelet effect of clopidogrel. Mol Biol Rep. 2019;46:4195-9.

104. Saiz-Rodríguez M, Belmonte C, Caniego JL, Koller D, Zubiaur P, Bárcena E, et al. Influence of CYP450 Enzymes, CES1, PON1, ABCB1, and P2RY12 polymorphisms on clopidogrel response in patients subjected to a percutaneous neurointervention. Clin Ther. 2019;41:1199-212.

105. Laizure SC, Hu ZY, Potter PM, Parker RB. Inhibition of carboxylesterase-1 alters clopidogrel metabolism and disposition. Xenobiotica. 2020;50:245-51.

106. Neuvonen M, Tarkiainen EK, Tornio A, Hirvensalo P, Tapaninen T, Paile-Hyvärinen M, et al. Effects of genetic variants on carboxylesterase 1 gene expression, and clopidogrel pharmacokinetics and antiplatelet effects. Basic Clin Pharmacol Toxicol. 2018;122:341-5.

107. Mirzaev KB, Osipova DV, Kitaeva EJ, Shprakh VV, Abdullaev SP, Andreev DA, et al. Effects of the rs2244613 polymorphism of the CES1 gene on the antiplatelet effect of the receptor P2Y12 blocker clopidogrel. Drug Metab Pers Ther. 2019;34(3):20180039.

108. Mansour A, Bachelot-Loza C, Nesseler N, Gaussem P, Gouin-Thibault I. P2Y12 inhibition beyond thrombosis: effects on inflammation. Int J Mol Sci. 2020;21:E1391.

109. Kim KA, Song WG, Lee HM, Joo HJ, Park JY. Effect of P2Y1 and P2Y12 genetic polymorphisms on the ADP-induced platelet aggregation in a Korean population. Thromb Res. 2013;132:221-6.

110. Fontana P, Dupont A, Gandrille S, Bachelot-Loza C, Reny JL, Aiach M, et al. Adenosine diphosphate-induced platelet aggregation is associated with P2Y12 gene sequence variations in healthy subjects. Circulation. 2003;108:989-95.

111. Li JL, Fu Y, Qin SB, Liang GK, Liu J, Nie XY, et al. Association between P2RY12 gene polymorphisms and adverse clinical events in coronary artery disease patients treated with clopidogrel: A systematic review and meta-analysis. Gene. 2018;657:69-80.

112. Li X, Jiang L, Sun S, Li W, Li X, Miao Z, et al. The influence of ABCB1 and P2Y12 genetic variants on clinical outcomes in Chinese intracranial artery stenosis patients. Clin Exp Pharmacol Physiol. 2018;45:978-82.

113. Nie XY, Li JL, Zhang Y, Xu Y, Yang XL, Fu Y, et al. Haplotype of platelet receptor P2RY12 gene is associated with residual clopidogrel on-treatment platelet reactivity. J Zhejiang Univ Sci B. 2017;18:37-47.

114. Zhao K, Yang M, Lu Y, Sun S, Li W, Li X, et al. P2Y12 polymorphisms and the risk of adverse clinical events in patients treated with clopidogrel: a meta-analysis. Drug Res (Stuttg). 2019;69:23-31.

115. Ulehlova J, Slavik L, Kucerova J, Krcova V, Vaclavik J, Indrak K. Genetic polymorphisms of platelet receptors in patients with acute myocardial infarction and resistance to antiplatelet therapy. Genet Test Mol Biomarkers. 2014;18:599-604.

116. Siasos G, Oikonomou E, Vavuranakis M, Kokkou E, Mourouzis K, Tsalamandris S, et al. Genotyping, platelet activation, and cardiovascular outcome in patients after percutaneous coronary intervention: two pieces of the puzzle of clopidogrel resistance. Cardiology. 2017;137:104-13.

117. Su J, Zheng N, Li Z, Huangfu N, Mei L, Xu X, et al. Association of GCK gene DNA methylation with the risk of clopidogrel resistance in acute coronary syndrome patients. J Clin Lab Anal. 2020;34:e23040.

118. Sukmawan R, Hoetama E, Suridanda Danny S, Giantini A, Listiyaningsih E, Gilang Rejeki V, et al. Increase in the risk of clopidogrel resistance and consequent TIMI flow impairment by DNA hypomethylation of CYP2C19 gene in STEMI patients undergoing primary percutaneous coronary intervention (PPCI). Pharmacol Res Perspect. 2021;9:e00738.

119. Krammer TL, Mayr M, Hackl M. microRNAs as promising biomarkers of platelet activity in antiplatelet therapy monitoring. Int J Mol Sci. 2020;21:3477.

120. Krammer TL, Kollars M, Kyrle PA, Hackl M, Eichinger S, Traby L. Plasma levels of platelet-enriched microRNAs change during antiplatelet therapy in healthy subjects. Front Pharmacol. 2022;13:1078722.

121. Conran N, Rees DC. Prasugrel hydrochloride for the treatment of sickle cell disease. Expert Opin Investig Drugs. 2017;26:865-72.

122. Alaoui MZ, Guy A, Khalki L, Limami Y, Benomar A, Zaid N, et al. Current antiplatelet agents, those under development and therapeutic targets. Med Sci (Paris). 2020;36:348-57.

123. Cavallari LH, Obeng AO. Genetic determinants of $P2Y_{12}$ inhibitors and clinical implications. Interv Cardiol Clin. 2017;6:141-9.

124. Bonney PA, Yim B, Brinjikji W, Walcott BP. Pharmacogenomic considerations for antiplatelet agents: the era of precision medicine in stroke prevention and neurointerventional practice. Cold Spring Harb Mol Case Stud. 2019;5:a003731.

125. Zhao Z, Wang Y, Tian N, Yan H, Wang J. Synthesis and biological evaluation of N 6 derivatives of 8-azapurine as novel antiplatelet agents. RSC Med Chem. 2021;12:1414-27.

126. Kabil MF, Abo Dena AS, El-Sherbiny IM. Ticagrelor. Profiles Drug Subst Excip Relat Methodol. 2022;47:91-111.

127. Sanderson NC, Parker WA, Storey RF. Ticagrelor: clinical development and future potential. Rev Cardiovasc Med. 2021;22:373-94.

128. He S, Lin Y, Tan Q, Mao F, Chen K, Hao J, et al. Ticagrelor resistance in cardiovascular disease and ischemic stroke. J Clin Med. 2023;12:1149.

129. Zhang X, Zhang X, Tong F, Cai Y, Zhang Y, Song H, et al. Gut microbiota induces high platelet response in patients with ST segment elevation myocardial infarction after ticagrelor treatment. eLife. 2022;11:e70240.

130. Foley SE, Tuohy C, Dunford M, Grey MJ, De Luca H, Cawley C, et al. Gut microbiota regulation of P-glycoprotein in the intestinal epithelium in maintenance of homeostasis. Microbiome. 2021;9:183.

131. Máchal J, Hlinomaz O. Efficacy of P2Y12 receptor blockers after myocardial infarction and genetic variability of their metabolic pathways. Curr Vasc Pharmacol. 2019;17:35-40.

132. Chen YC, Lin FY, Lin YW, Cheng SM, Chang CC, Lin RH, et al. Platelet microRNA 365-3p expression correlates with high on-treatment platelet reactivity in coronary artery disease patients. Cardiovasc Drugs Ther. 2019;33:129-37.

133. Laurent D, Dodd WS, Small C, Gooch MR, Ghosh R, Goutnik M, et al. Ticagrelor resistance: a case series and algorithm for management of non-responders. J Neurointerv Surg. 2022;14:179-83.

134. Eisert WG. Dipyridamole in antithrombotic treatment. Adv Cardiol. 2012;47:78-86.

135. Fontana P, Reny JL. Pharmacogenetics and antiplatelet drugs. Rev Med Interne. 2005;9:725-32.

136. Urano M, Kitahara M, Kishi K, Goto E, Tagami T, Fukami T, et al. Physical characteristics of cilostazol-hydroxybenzoic acid cocrystals prepared using a spray drying method. Crystals. 2020;10:313.

137. Kherallah RY, Khawaja M, Olson M, Angiolillo D, Birnbaum Y. Cilostazol: a review of basic mechanisms and clinical uses. Cardiovasc Drugs Ther. 2022;36:777-92.

138. de Havenon A, Sheth KN, Madsen TE, Johnston KC, Turan TN, Toyoda K, et al. Cilostazol for secondary stroke prevention: history, evidence, limitations, and possibilities. Stroke. 2021;52:e635-45.

139. Ikeda Y, Yamanouchi J, Kumon Y, Yasukawa M, Hato T. Association of platelet response to cilostazol with clinical outcome and CYP genotype in patients with cerebral infarction. Thromb Res. 2018;172:14-20.

140. Yokoyama T, Yamauchi S, Yamagata K, Kaneshiro Y, Urano Y, Murata K, et al. Impact of cilostazol pharmacokinetics on the development of cardiovascular side effects in patients with cerebral infarction. Biol Pharm Bull. 2021;44:1767-74.

141. Lee HI, Byeon JY, Kim YH, Lee CM, Choi CI, Jang CG, et al. Effects of CYP2C19 and CYP3A5 genetic polymorphisms on the pharmacokinetics of cilostazol and its active metabolites. Eur J Clin Pharmacol. 2018;74:1417-26.

142. Sharifi-Rad J, Sharopov F, Ezzat SM, Zam W, Ademiluyi AO, Oyeniran OH, et al. An updated review on glycoprotein IIb/IIIa inhibitors as antiplatelet agents: basic and clinical perspectives. High Blood Press Cardiovasc Prev. 2023;30:93-107.

143. Floyd CN, Ferro A. The PlA1/A2 polymorphism of glycoprotein IIIa in relation to efficacy of antiplatelet drugs: a systematic review and meta- analysis. Br J Clin Pharmacol. 2014;77:446-57.

144. O'Connor FF, Shields DC, Fitzgerald A, Cannon CP, Braunwald E, Fitzgerald DJ. Genetic variation in glycoprotein IIb/IIIa (GPIIb/IIIa) as a determinant of the responses to an oral GPIIb/IIIa antagonist in patients with unstable coronary syndromes. Blood. 2001;98:3256-60.

145. Morrison JT, Govsyeyev N, Hess CN, Bonaca MP. Vorapaxar for prevention of major adverse cardiovascular and limb events in peripheral artery disease. J Cardiovasc Pharmacol Ther. 2022;27:1-5.

146. Anderson MS, Kosoglou T, Statkevich P, Li J, Rotonda J, Meehan AG, Cutler DL. No pharmacokinetic drug-drug interaction between prasugrel and vorapaxar following multiple-dose administration in healthy volunteers. Clin

Pharmacol Drug Dev. 2018;7:143-50.

147. Li Z, Gnatenko DV, Bahou WF. Platelet Genomics. In: Gresele P, Kleiman NS, Lopez JA, Page CP, editors. Platelets in thrombotic and non-thrombotic disorders: pathophysiology, pharmacology and therapeutics: an Update. Cham: Springer; 2017.p.213-26.

148. Arachiche A, Nieman MT. The Platelet PARs. In: Gresele P, Kleiman NS, Lopez JA, Page CP, editors. Platelets in thrombotic and non- thrombotic disorders: pathophysiology, pharmacology and therapeutics: an Update. Cham: Springer; 2017.p.171-85.

149. Castrichini M, Luzum JA, Pereira N. Pharmacogenetics of antiplatelet therapy. Annu Rev Pharmacol Toxicol. 2023;63:211-29.

150. Pereira NL, Rihal C, Lennon R, Marcus G, Shrivastava S, Bell MR, et al. Effect of CYP2C19 genotype on ischemic outcomes during oral P2Y12 inhibitor therapy: a meta-analysis. JACC Cardiovasc Interv. 2021;14:739-50.

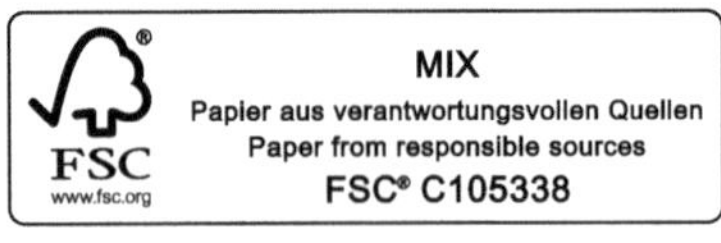

Printed by Books on Demand GmbH, Norderstedt / Germany